Dear Katherine -

Just to remind you of life in NYC - even though it wasn't like before.

Love -

Alec

11-10-22

JOURNAL OF THE PLAGUE YEARS

APRIL 2020 TO APRIL 2022

ALEC PRUCHNICKI MD

Journal of the Plague Years
April 2020 to April 2022

Published in the United States

Print ISBN: 978-1-66786-476-1
eBook ISBN: 978-1-66786-477-8

INTRODUCTION

The account of the Covid pandemic you are about to read is unlike any you have ever seen in the mainstream media. It is a compilation of almost 500 posts done mostly day to day during the plague in real time. These posts were usually done late at night after I reviewed the events of that day and so were written when I was tired, cranky, and sometimes a little drunk after a late-night party or dinner. They were never meant to be shown to the public but only to a small number of close friends, and so are filled with errors in spelling, punctuation, grammar, and capitalization, along with various computer glitches. Language purists and internet trolls will have a field day with these errors. But rather than clean up the numerous mistakes and run the risk of changing the content, I've left everything as heart felt as the nights I wrote them.

The only changes I have made have been to attempt to avoid political censorship algorithms that might inhibit publication and publicity. So, our presidents become T**** and B****, our former governor is C****, our former mayor D*******, the political parties are the D******** and R**********, and those opposed to the vaccine are anti-v******. I hope this works.

There are also many predictions, both accurate and inaccurate, trivial observations, and just plan errors of fact that I made at the time. I did the best I could with the knowledge I had. But in spite of all these problems, maybe some of these observations will be of benefit to someone somewhere. That is why these subjective observations made by just one individual are being presented to the public. I hope it helps.

Alec Pruchnicki MD

April 1, 2020

Journal of the Plague Year, day one. Other people are doing this, but maybe my perspective as a health care provider might help. I'm not on the very front lines, the docs, nurses and therapists inside the hospital are. My practice is in an assisted living facility, 127 residents, in the heart of New York City. They are old (68-102 years old), sick, mostly poor (we're supported by NY Medicaid), and multi-racial. We've done a lot to control the virus that I'll describe in future posts. Meanwhile, although I've been a Facer for over a year, I'm not good on FB methods, so if you see something interesting or relevant share it for me. A billion people on FB, so there's got to be someone somewhere who would benefit from what I'll be saying. See you again soon.

Journal of the Plague Year, day 2. the ALF residents where I work have been effected. When we were notified that one of our residents who was in the hospital for a different reason, was positive for COVID, the facility went on lock down. All group activities stopped (dining room, exercise classes, nightly movie, activity room, library, etc). The residents were told to stay in their rooms on isolation, and almost all complied even though we have no enforcement mechanism. Meds and meals were brought to them individually so nobody missed any meals or doses of meds. Fortunately, at our place everyone has their own studio apartment, no shared apartments. So, individual isolation was possible. More tomorrow. My temp today 98.2

Journal of the Plague Year, day 3. The effect of the ALF lock down on on residents. Most stayed in their rooms with TV, radio, books to keep them busy and phones and internet for contact with outside family and friends, all of whom were banned from visiting the facility. A few of the demented residents still went up to the dining room or down to the medication room (called "The Wellness Center") and had to be redirected. A few anxious or depressed ones got more anxious and depressed. A few confused ones got more confused, sometimes by a lot. But now the isolation is eased up a little. More on that tomorrow. My temp today 97.8

Journal of the Plague Year, Day 4. The ALF where I work is starting to ease up just a little on isolation. Our last known exposure was about 2 weeks ago with no new exposures, so we think it is about as safe as we can determine, at least with the tools we have now. Patients still get meds and meals delivered to their rooms individually but they are allowed to come out as long as they don't congregate with each other. The physical and occupational therapists are back in the building and starting to see patients again in one on one sessions. We need to reverse the debility people have experience from sitting in their rooms all day. A few people have left the building for a few hours, although we are trying to discourage too much of that. Still no visitors entering the building. The exercise class has bee broken up so that instead of one group of 25 in one room with have 4 groups of 6-7 in the hallways sitting on chairs that are spaced 6 feet apart. Let's hope no new cases occur so we can continue and expand this instead of having to resume isolation. Tomorrow, the effect on staff. temp today is 97.8

Journal of the Plague Year, Day 5 (4/5/20). When we went into lock down because of the two cases of COVID, the staff had to adjust. Everyone, including myself, has their temperature checked as soon as they come in the door, and the temp is entered into a computer for future tracking. All contacts between any staff member and resident requires a mask and gloves for the staffer. this, plus individual deliveries of meds and meals slows everything down a lot, but so far every resident has gotten everything they should get. There have been some indication of stress on the staff, but also measures to address the stress. More on that tomorrow. Temp today 98.0

Journal of the Plague Year, Day 6. Some of the staff have been staying home because of feeling sick (colds, coughs, or just general malaise) so others have to step up with extra hours. Everything is getting done, but with more effort. The facility is now providing lunch every day so staff won't leave the building and also as a little perk for dedicated workers. They say you shouldn't eat as an emotional reward, but that's ridiculous. Of course people eat as an emotional reward, and especially now. Tomorrow, the nurses. temp today 97.8.

Journal of the Plague Year, Day 7. The nurses at our ALF are the most exposed to risk. The personal care assistants (PCAs) each have a panel of 20-25 patients during the day and the PCAs at night float from floor to floor. The nurses have to deliver meds to all the 127 residents. We have several LPNs (licensed practical nurses) who are full time, a few agency nurses (temporary hires) and barely enough. Even our CEO, who is a nurse, was distributing meds, which is way way below her pay grade. Everyone is masked and gloved but there can always be accidents. The DOH (Department of Health) has issued guidelines for nursing home quarantine procedures and it turns out we are following them, more or less. This is a lot for an ALF, but I think it helps. We were notified of our third COVID positive patient, who is in the hospital, but 3 out of 127 isn't too bad, unless there are more hidden cases. Tomorrow, the effect on the city. temp today 98.0

Journal of the Plague Year, Day 8. Outside of my ALF and its residents and staff the world has changed too. I live in Greenwich Village which is usually a neighborhood with a busy night life of restaurants, bar, and theaters. Not now. All of the bars and theaters are closed, and most of the restaurants. Some restaurants are open and doing a brisk take out business, but I'm not sure it will be enough to tide them over until this is done. All the pharmacies, and a few of the groceries and bodegas are also open. The supermarkets were swamped with panic buying, hoarding and long lines at the start of this, but now things are back to normal and everyone is well stocked. There should be no trouble getting essentials like food, medications, and red wine. Fresh Direct and the other home delivery companies are also swamped and booked up for weeks, so supermarkets are much more convenient. Tomorrow COVID, race, and the subways. temp today 97.9.

Journal of the Plague Year, Day 9. Lots of reports from all over the country of higher COVID death rates among blacks. Some is poverty, pre-existing medical conditions, poor access to med care, and even rumors in the black community that blacks can't get COVID. Let me add one more observation: the subways. I take the seventh avenue express 2 and 3 trains to and from work every day. before the quarantine, the people taking the train, at least from 96th to 14th street, were pretty much multi-racial with large numbers of white, black, hispanic and asian riders of all ages. since the lock down the total numbers of riders has gone down a lot, but now the remaining riders are overwhelmingly black and hispanic, and not as many very young students or very old people. The most likely explanation is that these are the people who work at low paying service jobs with little job security, little direct contact with others (can't do their jobs over the internet), and can't afford taxis and Ubers to get to work. Not only are they at risk, but when they go back to their communities they increase the potential spread of the virus there. I've seen little data on hispanic rates, so we'll have to see if that mirrors black disease rates. temp today 99.0

Journal of the Plague Year, Day 10. Let me digress a little from my own experiences and address some medical issues, since I am after all, a doctor. Lots of information has been coming out about cures/treatments. Chloroquin has been pushed as a possible treatment or prevention. The New York Department of Health (DOH) has issued guidelines saying that it can be used for symptomatic patients who have already tested positive for COVID. Not only shouldn't it be used for prevention but it has issued orders to physicians and pharmacists not to prescribe it for anyone else except for Lupus patients and a few others who were taking it before. Choroquin is needed by these patients, but has side effects and can kill you if it's not needed. Repeat, it can kill you, so don't fuck around with it until it is proven to work. In general, listen to anything said by Dr. Fauci, the Center for Disease Control (CDC), or your state DOH. Don' listen to ANYTHING said by President T****. temp today 98.0

Journal of the Plague Year, Day 11. Today is Holy Saturday. This is the day my mom died in 2008. Not April 11 but March 22, one of the earliest Easters in a century. I never remember the date but always remember Holy Saturday. I also never get depressed over it, just sentimental. She had advanced Alzheimer's and no quality of life. If her younger self had been able to see her condition, I'm sure she would have said "that's no way to live," which she often used to describe other terminal family members. As long as we're on a morbid theme, one more fact. I've started to make out my will. I'm really good at procrastinating and should have done this years ago under much less dramatic circumstances. But, I could never figure out how to divide a West Village Co-op among 15 or so relatives and charities. Now my executor will have to figure it out. Tomorrow; cancellations from conventions to Burning Man. temp today 97.8

Journal of the Plague Year, Day 12, Easter Sunday, April 12, 2020. Normally, Easter is time to get together for large religious services or large family meals. Not now. But there have been other group activities that have been cancelled and we sometimes manage to make due. I attend the America Medical Directors Association convention most years, and planned to go to Chicago for this years'. It was cancelled, but will be presented on-line in a few weeks. The American Geriatrics Society in Long Beach was cancelled with no further plans at this time. So one adapted and one didn't. The Gerontological Society of America plans to meet in Philadelphia in November. We'll see. These meetings are chances to meet with colleagues from around the country, hear what is happening, and take a few days break from routine to reinvigorate. Eventually these will resume, but not just yet. thousands of people in one room won't do right now. Tomorrow, local meetings cancelling and coping. Temp today 98.0

Journal of the Plague Year, Day 13. I described medical conventions that were cancelled. But, some meetings have managed to cope. My political club, the Village Independent D********, cancelled two face to face meetings in March and replaced them with virtual meetings using something called Cisco. The meetings were a little difficult to get used to, but we managed to make all the decisions we needed eventually. A single payer advocacy group, Physicians for a National Health Program, NY Metro Chapter, also had two virtual meetings which got most things done that had to be done using Zoom. There are ways of getting some business done over the internet, but it will take time to get used to them. Several administrators at my ALF are now working from home fairly successfully. Some meetings might be more difficult. Tomorrow, virtual Burning Man. temp today 99.1.

Journal of the Plague Year, Day 14. Some cancelled events are more difficult to put on line than others. I've been to Burning Man five times, but missed the last few years. But, this year I had everything set up. Nothing could go wrong. I had my RV reserved in Oakland, a good inside track to get tickets and, most importantly, someone to cover my two weeks away from my medical practice. The 70,000 people arts fair/party in the Nevada wasteland north of Reno was a done deal. Then came March, COVID and a few days ago, cancellation. The loss of a big party is not the worse thing that will result from this pandemic. But, I wonder how it will play out. There are many creative artistic people involved in BM and lots of them should know how to make artistic, creative, enjoyable videos to replace the Burn. The number of fire dancers alone should fill up a week of videos. More seriously, political conventions, elections and the rest of the country needs to be organized. His Majesty King Donald the First thinks he can do it. I'll take the fire dancers. temp today 98.4.

Journal of the Plague Year, Day 15. More meetings and services are being done remotely, and we're getting ready for some of this at the ALF where I work. I've been healthy so far, and have gotten into work without a problem. But anyone with a temperature or signs of a respiratory infection (cough with or without sputum, nasal congestion, sore throat, shortness of breath, high temperature) is told to go home for 7-14 days after the symptoms are gone. I've set up some remote links so that if this happens to me I can still remote in and renew prescriptions or order new medications. The nurses at the facility would have to examine the patient, let me know what they find, and then I can order any tests, meds, hospital transfers, etc, over the phone. this isn't the best way to practice medicine, but it's a back up if needed. Maybe even ZOOM if I can learn it well enough. I'm hoping I won't need it. temp today 97.8.

Journal of the Plague Year, Day 16. there is a lot of information out in the media and on the internet about what is happening and where. but there is also a lot of missing information. In nyc there have been stories about individual communities like New Rochelle and some individual nursing homes, but I can't find info on nursing homes and assisted living facilities in general. there is usually a gossip grapevine of ALF and nursing home directors who trade information unofficially, but this has shut down as much as I can determine. nobody is saying anything about their own facilities, at least at this time. Maybe the data isn't there, maybe they don't want attention on them, even unofficially, unless everyone comes out simultaneously. the state department of health or maybe federal Medicare program might eventually show the data since they have the power to collect it, but not just yet. we don't know what we don't know. temp today 97.6.

Journal of the Plague Year, Day 17. Had a happy hour tonight over Zoom. 6 friends from graduate school having drinks, talking and seeing each other face to face, sort of. No hacking by outsiders. I guess we need to get used to this for the time being. I've also been on Zoom for meetings but this was the first time I discovered my lap top's built in microphone along with the built in camera that makes this possible. No earth shaking significance here, or lessons to be learned about the pandemic, just a few friends getting together. We'll do this again. temp today 97.6

Journal of the Plague Year, Day 18. Many nursing homes and ALFs are on lock down and visitors are banned or discouraged. Family members and friends of residents at these facilities are frantic because they don't have direct access to their loved one and have complained about the lack of information and transparency from these facilities. But there is a reason for this, and not an ominous or sneaky one. Every minute a provider (doctor, nurse, social worker, etc) spends on the phone speaking to family is a minute away from the patients who need us. We would love to communicate more, but it's not so easy. When I speak to families, I can't just give a few seconds "your mom is ok" message. There is usually a discussion of details, plans for the future, problems at the facility etc. In the 5-10-15 minutes on the phone I can see another patient who might need me. When we are all stretched to the limit in terms of time, this is a problem. So, when staff aren't as communicative as people would like, please cut us a little slack. We are doing the best we can with the time we have. temp today 98.2

Journal of the Plague Year, Day 19, Sunday April 19th. Masks? Masks?! We don't need no stinkin' masks! Both last Sunday and today when I went out for my morning bagel and coffee I noticed a lot of people not wearing masks, here in Greenwich Village. Often it was couples walking together. I guess they assume that since they're together all the time, whatever infection they spread to each other will be inevitable. How this effects infections to and from other people on the street isn't so clear. Today I did a count and there were about 61 people I passed wearing masks, including me, and 28 not. A few couples, some joggers, dog walkers and bike riders made up the maskless group. If I remember, I'll try to do this on upcoming Sundays and see if there is a trend. temp today 98.2

Journal of the Plague Year, Day 20. A lot of front page stories have come out about CORVID deaths in nursing homes with some horrific cases, like the NH in Jersey that had 17 bodies piled up in their morgue. You can do an internet search for "New York State Nursing Home Deaths" and get a list from the NY Health Department of all nursing homes with more than 5 deaths. But, there's something strange about it. Some of the best nursing homes still have a lot of deaths. Mary Manning Walsh NH in Manhattan has 32 deaths listed, the most in the borough. But MMW has always been considered one of the best, if not the best, nursing home in Manhattan. So, why so many deaths? Is it because they have hospice beds with terminal patients? Maybe because they are good they take in sicker patients. Maybe our criteria for what is a "good" nursing home is wrong. After this is over I hope some state or federal agency does a careful retrospective analysis of what caused these deaths and what could the nursing homes have done, if anything, to prevent them. temp today 98.0

Journal of the Plague Year, Day 21. Typhoid Mary Mallon was a cook who worked in the mansions of wealthy families in the early 1900s. wherever she worked typhoid fever broke out and eventually a writer tracked her down and publicized her story. she never had typhoid herself but was an asymptomatic carrier who caused the infection of over 50 people and the deaths of at least two. she was in and out of involuntary isolation on North Brother Island hospital, about 26 years total, and that's where she died. We know that CORVID can be carried by asymptomatic carriers. We don't know how many cases are carried by these individuals and how many are carried by people who have, or eventually develop, symptoms. the outbreaks in Washington nursing homes, or in New Rochelle were, I think, both started with one person. One asymptomatic person can do a lot of damage and we don't know how many of them are out there. that's why we need testing of a lot of people. Tomorrow-about these tests. temp today 97.2

Journal of the Plague Year, Day 22. The ALF where I work is now up to 6 residents and one staff member. None of the 6 residents had obvious upper respiratory symptoms. It's not clear how the ERs they were in picked up on COVID. Were there minor symptoms that we didn't see and the ER did? Three are in rehab, two back at the facility on isolation, one died from probably unrelated causes. One staff member also is positive and her main symptom was a temp. she is at home on isolation for up to 14 days. If this is at all representative of what's happening around the city, it means that the vast majority of COVID infected people are asymptomatic and might be spreading the virus without even realizing it. This is one of the reasons testing is needed so that positive people can be identified and go on isolation quickly and not after spreading the bug around. But testing isn't that easy to get. When it is easy I'll let people know on these posts, but not just yet. temp today 98.2

Journal of the Plague Year, Day 23. some testing has been done of the general population to see how many have antibodies to COVID19. It's not 100% sure that these antibodies indicate complete immunity to a new infection, or to symptoms arriving at a later date, or even if all the tests are accurate. But, just for the sake of argument let's say the tests do indicate 100% immunity and lack of antibodies indicates 100% susceptibility to catching the virus. Santa Clara in California had about 4% antibody positive and NYC about 20%. That still means that if the virus has a second wave because of natural progression of the pandemic or because we lighten up restrictions too early there will be lots of people who can come down with it. 80% of NYC will be open to infection which possibly means we can have a second wave much worse than the first. And, if the second wave comes in during the fall flu season we will have people sick and dying from the flu at the same time they are sick and dying from COVID. Better testing in the next few months can help us track disease progression, but whether we track or not there are a lot of people out there who could still catch it. Sorry to be so gloomy. I'll try and find something more positive tomorrow. temp today 98.2

Journal of Plague Year, Day 24. A lot of people have been talking about the need for wide spread testing for CORVID to get the pandemic under control and start to open up society. But, there is a problem. When I started to do my clinical clerkships in medical school where I actually started seeing patients, the senior attending physicians would often tell us, "Don't order a test unless you know what you're going to do with it." Ordering a test just to satisfy your curiosity would cause problems if you found something you didn't need to know but now had to pursue just because it looked fishy. That led to more tests, more treatments, etc. So, with CORVID testing, if we test and find uninfected people, asymptomatic infected people, symptomatic infected people, or those who had the virus and are now through it what do we do? The most difficult next step is contact tracing which is very time consuming. But what do we do with contact tracing once we find an infected person? The answer is to put him/her on isolation for 14 days to see if he becomes symptomatic and thus can infect others. At my alf, we don't have tests so we just skipped ahead to the last step: isolation. Residents were isolated in their rooms for about two weeks and monitored closely for symptoms. Staff temperatures were check every day as soon as we entered the building and any temp over 100 or respiratory symptoms meant the person went home for 14 days. We think that may have helped us keep our infection rate down, but who knows. We could still be missing a lot. More details tomorrow. These posts are getting longer and longer, but I hope not too boring. temp today 97.8

Journal of the Plague Year, Day 25. Some states and cities are starting to open up. There are even some signs here in the city. The subways during rush hour have about a half dozen people, including homeless sleeping on the seats, instead of one or two. Cars on the streets are going up a little and I now actually have to look when crossing. One of the three neighborhood Starbucks has opened for take out orders. Fresh Direct is delivering to me tomorrow night, the first time in a month. These are all pretty much grasping at straws in the hope that these moves won't increase infections. We might know if these moves were premature in about 3 weeks, or maybe not until the fall. We'll see. temp today 98.4

Journal of the Plague Year, Day 26, Sunday April 26, 2020. To my T**** supporting friends and relatives (yes, I do have T**** supporting friends and relatives) don't take offense at what I am about to say. Don't listen to ANYTHING he says on health care issues. By accident and statistical probability he might accidentally say something accurate now and then, but the chances of that are pretty low. Listen to the doctors and health care experts and remember to read between the lines when they have to phrase their comments in the least direct way possible so as not to upset him. temp today 98.9

Journal of the Plague Year, Day 27. I mentioned before that a lot of people, maybe about a third, are not wearing masks out on the street. It seemed to me that a lot of these were young couples, but I wasn't sure if I was right. I spoke to a friend who lives in the suburbs of Maryland where there are a lot of open spaces to wander around without violating the 6 foot space. She also mentioned that she saw a lot of young couples without masks, so maybe it's not just my imagination. the last three days I actually did a count on the streets in my neighborhood just looking at couples. There were 19 with no masks at all, 24 couples with both people masked, and 9 with one person masked and one not. Most were young, but not all. I don't know if this indicates couples, young or otherwise, are dumber, healthier, more confident or what. the significance is yet to be determined, if there is any significance in this. temp today 99.2

Journal of the Plague Year, Day 28. I've described how we do things at the ALF where I work. Lots of isolation, no outside visitors, leaving the building only when absolutely necessary. we don't have testing at our place so we skipped ahead to isolation for lots of people. We had another resident go into the ER for an unrelated matter and ended up testing positive. The Sinai ER is testing almost everyone, if not everyone, who comes in for almost anything. At the ALF we are adding another rule that anyone who goes to the ER for any reason and is treated and sent back to us goes on isolation for 14 days, even if there was no testing, rather than take a chance. Of all the people who went to the ER and tested positive, none went in for respiratory symptoms. So we are still assuming there is a vast number of asymptomatic carriers. Eventually, if testing becomes widely available we can start to test everyone and see what the rate of asymptomatic healthy older adults at our place really is. But when testing is that available is unknown. Just today in a carefully worded statement Fauci said he hopes there will be a significant increase in testing. We'll see. temp today 99.2

Journal of the Plague Year, Day 29. Things sometimes move fast in the middle of an emergency. Two weeks ago I wrote an article for my neighborhood newspaper Westview News. I talked about several research projects being done by Northwell medical system, and one of them was on an anti-viral drug called remdesivir. Today Dr. Fauci mentions a study which shows that this same drug shortens the time it takes for people with CORVID to recover from 14 days to 11 and might also improve the death rate from 11% down to 8%. Normally you don't change medical care just because of one study. You want the results to be duplicated in another study by another group. But in an emergency like this, this one study is going to have a major impact and it remdesivir will be the standard of care. I can imagine my own patients and their families asking for this by tomorrow morning and I'll have to tell them no, at least for now. I have to see the actual study and then see if it is relevant for my patients, who are not symptomatic. We'll see. temp today 98.5

Journal of the Plague Year, Day 30. Lots of newspaper articles about homeless people in the subways. there always were a lot, especially late night, and the general number of people living in the subways has been about 2000 for a few years. Recently, more are around in the daytime where they can be seen by the media and also some my be more psychotic as stress takes its toll. I seem to have seen more psychotic behavior recently, but I wasn't sure and so didn't mention it. Now the cops are moving in and homeless are being given the choice of hospital or homeless shelter, but they can't stay on the subway. This is a version of the closing round announcement at bars, "You don't have to go home but you can't stay here." The subways will even be completely closed from 1 AM to 5 or 6 AM for a complete cleaning, the first time I ever remember the subways being closed. The problem of homelessness has been one the city and country has been unable to solve, but able to avoid looking at. Now we can't avoid looking, it's right in front of us. No new money for housing yet, but we'll see. temp today 98.4

Journal of the Plague Year, Day 31. I wasn't sure what to write today until I took my usual after dinner nap and was woken up by cheering and banging at 7 PM. The cheering that people are doing to acknowledge the work of first responders is very appreciated and heartening. As I've mentioned before, I'm not a front line responder, but maybe a third line responder (hospitals-first, nursing homes-second, assisted living-third). I found a way to show appreciation of the nurses in my ALF; chocolate. Applause is good, chocolate is better. Within my budget I'll see how much of this I can do in the future. Saving lives builds up an appetite. temp today 98.4

Journal of the Plague Year, Day 32. when I talk about the docs in the hospital being on the front line, I'm drawing from some of my old experience. I haven't taken care of hospital patients for a long time, but what I remember of being a Resident and later an Attending, the death of any patient brought out soul searching and a mental post mortem of the case. What did I miss? What could I have done differently? Would this other treatment have helped better? That's for one case. I can't imagine what's happening to the docs now who are losing case after case. It must be a horror. But, you go on, usually. One recent suicide of a doc who worked in the ER is a warning to some of the others to find a way to relieve the stress of seeing all this around them. Good luck to them all. tempt today 98.0

Journal of the Plague Year, Day 33, Sunday May 3. It was a beautiful day today, 68 degrees, no humidity or rain. I went across from my building to the Hudson River Park, which is a narrow park with grass, bike lane and beautiful view of the river. Lots of people, some with masks, some without. Many couples without masks, just like I saw previously. A few cops were around but I didn't see them breaking up groups or ticketing anyone. If it weren't for the pandemic and people with masks it would look roughly like any other nice spring Sunday. I don't know if that's good, because we are getting back to normal, or bad because we're getting sloppy when it comes to precautions like masks and distance. We'll find out in a few weeks if we start to get a bump in cases or if we continue to go down in numbers. temp today 99.1

Journal of the Plague Year, Day 34. All this opening up of isolation is making me nervous. A little has been happening in NYC and I've described a little in some of these accounts. But what other states are doing is much worse. They are relaxing isolation while their numbers are still going up, without know how bad the infection rates are going to get. I thought NYC's experience would be a guide to these other states and our numbers, both good and bad, and our policies, both effective and ineffective, could be used by other states to help them plan their own policies. Since some of these states are rushing ahead with loosening up isolation it might work that their results for better or worse can be used as a guide for us. It's very little consolation for us in NYC to point to Texas or Florida and see what they're doing wrong and what we're doing right. There is enough death going around to produce misery in all of these states simultaneously. temp today 98.4

Journal of the Plague Year, Day 35. Tonight the subways shut down from 1 AM to 5 AM to do a careful cleaning. But the news might have gotten out already. Today for the first time in a while, there were no homeless people on the subway during each rush hour. The subway cars were pretty empty, but no obvious homeless people or even people begging, which is also unusual. I don't know where these people are going or how they are being taken care of, but at least for this one day things looked empty. we'll see how long this lasts. temp today 98.2

Journal of the Plague Year, Day 36. Things at work are falling into a routine. Patients who went to the ER, or Rehab, or an Urgent Care office (sometimes referred to as a doc-in-the-box) come back and are on isolation for two weeks. Meals and meds are still delivered and the staff all seems to have and use protective equipment whenever necessary. This routine doesn't indicate that the end of our precautions is at hand. More like "… this is not the beginning of the end, but perhaps the end of the beginning." which is what Churchill said during the early stage of WWII. Let's hope so. temp today 99.2

Journal of the Plague Year, Day 37. There was a piece on the news tonight about a "Miracle" patient from Jersey who was on a vent for two weeks and recovered even when his doctors thought he would die. This wasn't a miracle. It happens all the time. Patients who looked like they were dying recover and healthy ones die. Doctors can do everything wrong for a patient and he still recovers and likewise do everything right and some unforeseen event kills him. I wish we were as good at prediction as people, and some doctors, think we are. But, we're not. temp today 98.7

Journal of the Plague Year, Day 38. Well, our luck couldn't last forever. We had 7 documented patients with CORVID, six are ok and one died probably from unrelated causes. Today we got our 8th cases and first probable CORVID death. She had been slowly getting more debilitated and inactive over the last few days, but no clear respiratory symptoms, or even an elevated temperature. Two days ago she was found unresponsive in her apartment, sent to the ER and intubated immediately, which is often the protocol. She was tested for CORVID and was positive and this morning she died. Eventually we will get the death certificate and see if they list CORVID as one of the causes or if they just use the general catch all term of "cardiopulmonary arrest". As I mentioned previously, an unexpected death usually triggers a detailed looking back, an autopsy of the medical record. What did we miss? What could we have done differently? We haven't found any egregious errors, but there's always a doubt in the back of your mind. I hope I don't have to repeat this too many times in the coming months. temp today 98.4

Journal of the Plague Year, Day 39. I can't figure out how this outbreak makes people act so strange. When it started people were flocking to the supermarkets to stock up on food, especially chicken, paper towels and toilet paper. Toilet paper?! That stage has passed but for several weeks now I noticed there was a shortage of Cascade dish washer powder. My local D'Agostino's, Rite Aide, and Fresh Direct delivery all carried Cascade but all have been completely out of stock for several weeks. Are all these people stuck in their homes washing their dishes more frequently? This has been going on for weeks. Yesterday, for the first time, there were two boxes of Cascade on the shelf of my local D'Agostino's so I bought one and it will probably last about a year. What's next? temp today 98.4

Journal of the Plague Year, Day 40, Mother's Day Sunday May 10. More grasping at straws in hopes of a revival. Another pastry shop on Hudson street reopened today, and what's more they had a few customers waiting on line. Opening businesses won't mean anything unless customers come out and patronize those places.

A digression on Mother's Day. For my mom, Mother's Day wasn't a big thing. Her birthday was in early May, so she would get a big present then (or at least as big as I could afford) and a box of candy on Mother's Day (Loft's TV Mix). We never went out for dinner since my Mom was always so critical of the restaurants, even on Arthur Avenue with great places to eat. Growing up in the Great (but probably not the only) Depression she always thought the prices were too high. "They're charging how much for THIS." She was also critical of the food. She wasn't a great cook, spending her whole adult life working, but her mom, my Neapolitan grandma, and my dad were great cooks, so we always ate well. Too well. "We could get better at home." So, no Mom's day dinners. But, she did love that candy. Happy Mom's Day to all you Facers posting today. temp today. 97.8

Journal of the Plague Year, Day 41. I wasn't sure if I would write about the problems with testing for the virus, or new guidelines NY State has put forth for nursing home. But then I took my temperature with my old fashioned glass/mercury thermometer and it was 100.4. I wasn't too worried since my apartment gets very hot and that sometimes gives a false temperature. I shut the heat, opened the window and stuck the thermometer in my mouth to give it more time. But, it accidentally fell out and broke on the floor. At least I think it was accidental and not sabotage by some Monster from the Id (if you're not a boomer look it up). So, I'm not sure about my temperature. I feel ok, no symptoms, don't feel warm. If I'm still feeling ok, I'll go in tomorrow and they will take my temperature at the door. If it's high I'll try and find a place to test me and see if it's CORVID. If not, I have to find a drug store that has new thermometers in stock so I can keep track myself. I hope it's not, since there are a lot of people I came into contact with at work and tracking them is going to be a horror.

Journal of the Plague Year, Day 42. It looks like my temperature yesterday was probably a false alarm. Today when I went into work by temp was 97.4 and just now with a brand new digital thermometer it was 97.6. I was worried that a positive temp would require I be on isolation until I got a more accurate nasal test. But, it turns out the state is requiring all nursing homes and adult homes like mine test all staff members twice a week. This is going to be a real logistical pain to do, and maybe a physical pain as that swab gets closer to the brain, but it should give us some more accurate info. Needless to say, this mandate from the state comes without any funding, at least for now. I've brought home some codes and links to install in my home computer so that if I'm on isolation I can still do some of my medical work remotely. real (I hope) temp today 97.6

Journal of the Plague Year, Day 43. Starting last week the subways shut down at night from 1 AM to 5 AM. It was to do cleaning, get homeless people out of the subways and into shelters, hospitals, maybe empty hotels. Since then I've taken 10 subway rides going to and from work. The subway cars are much cleaner with almost no litter or spilled food/drink. There may have been only one possible homeless person riding the subway that I saw, although it was an imprecise guess. There has been only one person begging on the subway also. Both of these numbers are way down, even though the subways are completely open by rush hour. So, the cleaning at night is having some indirect effects. I don't know what happened to the homeless. Some newspaper articles have interviewed them and found some went to shelters, some to hospital ERs, and maybe a few to hotels which the city is paying for. This last point helps the homeless, helps the empty hotels, but might be expensive, although some of the shelters seem to be pretty expensive on a daily basis also. Ten subway rides isn't a lot. I'll let you know if the results change as we get a more statistically significant sample size. temp today 96.9, and this digital thermometer is much easier to use than the mercury one. I hope it's as accurate.

Journal of the Plague Year, Day 44. I was on a Zoom meeting with my political club, the Village Independent D******** which lasted almost 3 hours. I noticed something else, besides the length of the meeting. Several people had other meetings almost simultaneously. Some other meetings were before ours, some during ours, and some later and people had to leave us early. I hope this doesn't set too much of a precedent. If we are going to start double or triple scheduling meetings via Zoom then I can never use the excuse "...sorry, I have another meeting that night..." And before you say it, no this doesn't make retirement look more attractive, since these were all non-work meetings. On the other hand, I was able to attend while in my shorts and with a glass of wine in my hand, so maybe I can take 2 or 3 meetings a night. temp today 98.0

Journal of the Plague Year, Day 45. Sometimes even well meaning proposals to control this pandemic are easier said than done. C**** is mandating that all health care facilities for older adults (nursing homes and adult care facilities like mine) test their staff twice a week for the virus. this is a great idea and will help a lot except that we can't do it. One of the non-profit advocacy groups for ALFs estimated that it would mead 350,000 tests a week with an estimated cost of over $40 million, which would be over two billion dollars over a year. And that's assuming that the price doesn't go up once a shortage of test materials develops, which would happen almost immediately. I've heard that the state is providing 100,000 tests, but I haven't seen them yet. Many NH and ALF facilities operate on a shoestring budget and a big expense would either take resources that could be used for patient care, or even push a struggling facility into bankruptcy. Again, a great idea which would help us manage the virus a lot, but easier said than done. temp today 98.3

Journal of the Plague Year, Day 46. The CORVID count at our ALF is about 9. They all had one thing in common. None had clear respiratory symptoms but had the normal run of the mill problems you see in a population of this age. Some were just tired and lethargic, some had problems with falls, but none had clear coughing, sputum, runny nose, shortness of breath before they were sent to the ER. This is going to be a hard disease to track until we get universal testing. Also, many people who had respiratory symptoms, sometimes severe ones, didn't have CORVID. temp today 98.3

Addendum to Journal of the Plague Year. 9 PM tonight on channel 13, WNET educational station, "The Producers" with Zero Mostel and Gene Wilder. A little comic relief to take us back to the relatively good old days (1968!?) when Nazis were in a comedy and not the nightly news. It's 7, I hear cheering outside.

Journal of the Plague Year, Day 47, Sunday May 17. More restaurants and shops opening on Hudson street. Cowgirls Hall of Fame. Sweet Corner. But only for take out. This is probably a good thing if people don't get carried away. A rumor at Hudson Gourmet where I get my bacon egg and cheese roll was that everything is opening on May 26th, but I'm not sure if it's true. What worries me is pictures from the Jersey shore where some beaches opened and hundreds of people lined up with few face masks. People are eager to resume life, but maybe too eager. We'll find out in about 2-3 weeks after things open when the cases go up, and 2-3 weeks later when deaths go up. Let's hope the mask-less ones are right and all the doctors are wrong, but I don't think so. temp today 97.8

Journal of the Plague Year, Day 48. In the news today lots of talk about a new vaccine. A small study of 45 people had some promising results in terms of antibody production and safety. But, we will need larger numbers, even at this preliminary stage. Then the later stages of giving the vaccine to large numbers of people of all ages. It would be great if this could be done by the end of the year, but that is very unlikely. When a final study is set up with a control group and all the normal monitoring then we should all consider signing up. I will. temp today 97.5

Journal of the Plague Year, Day 49. Hydroxychloroquin is now getting more publicity since T**** claimed to be taking it. The NY Department of Health allows it to be used for people who already have COVID as a last desperate treatment. No COVID and docs are not supposed to prescribe it and pharmacies are not supposed to dispense it. And you don't want to cross the DOH since they can, if pissed off enough, pull your license. The medical literature generally says stay away from it for the time being. The studies don't support using it for treatment or prevention. There is one small VA study which showed that people who got hydroxychloroquin were twice as likely to die as people who didn't. It killed people. It can cause irregular heart beats which might be how it does it, but the numbers are usually very small. When this study was pointed out to T**** in a press conference his answer was that the VA doesn't like him much. In other words, he thinks those doctors doing the study were lying just to embarrass him. If he really is taking it, and people aren't sure about the honesty of his statements, then good luck to him. He might need it. temp today 98.3

Journal of the Plague Year, Day 50. The debate back and forth about when to open up has a lot of aspects to it, one of which is will people come out and patronize businesses that open even if they are allowed to. How scared people are about coming out will vary from location to location and business to business. This morning I got up a little late and got on the subway at 9:15 instead of 8:00. I was the only person in the car at 14th street, 34th street, 42nd street, 72nd street and 96th street. Not one other person during the 20 minute five stop trip. I don't know if this stark reminder of how much people are hiding out represents more behavior at more locations, but it may have shown that people aren't itching to get out as much as some people say. We'll see. temp today 98.6

Journal of the Plague Year, Day 51. At my job I got my first CORVID19 nasal swab test today. The state required all staff of nursing homes and adult homes to get tested twice a week. It provided the materials but the processing costs by the labs will have to be born by the institutions. This might be very expensive. My place has about 100 employees. Most, I think, have insurance and it may pay the processing costs which will help out the facility expenses. If a test is positive, the person has to stay away from work for two weeks and get retested with negative results before he can come back to work. I'll get my results on Tuesday the 26th. I'll let you know (or as we say in the Bronx, I'll let youse know). temp today 98.0

Journal of the Plague Year, Day 52. I saw on cable last night a vaccine specialist from Harvard who was talking about the chance of getting a vaccine. He was old and had white hair, so he probably knew what he was talking about. He said he was more worried about whether there would be a vaccine and not when there would be one. He pointed out that no disease that is transmitted through the nose has been eliminated by a vaccine. The movement of virus particles through the nasal membranes causes damage faster than antibodies, even those fortified with a vaccine, can neutralize them. Polio and Smallpox are the most successful cases of vaccine elimination and they are transmitted mostly by touch. Flu is inhaled but its vaccine is only about 50% effective and it has to be changed every year. I hope he's wrong, but this was a little unnerving. As a note added in proof, an anti malaria vaccine has been worked on for a century, and HIV vaccine for about 25 years, and neither are here yet. temp today 96.9

Journal of the Plague Year, Day 53. "I have discovered that all human evil comes from this, man's being unable to sit still in a room." Blaise Pascal 1623-1662. I don't know which 17th century calamity prompted Pascal to say this, but is seems to accurately describe a little of what is happening now. Every day now another place in The Village opens up for take out. Possibly there are also more people walking around in general. Churches all over the country opening up soon will add to this increased risk. We won't know if this will be inconsequential, a minor problem, or a major problem big enough to start a new mid-summer COVID wave. We'll know in about a month. temp today 97.7

Journal of the Plague Year, Day 54, Sunday May 24, 2020. Presumably to help out small restaurants, the city has allowed deliveries and take out meals to include alcohol. Besides regular meals, many small restaurants have used this to try and have some business during the lock down. They have started take out happy hours. Although you can't' go and sit in the restaurant or at the bar, you can come take out some food, if only the tiniest amount, and some alcohol with it. This afternoon, in the middle of beautiful weather, at 4 PM I went to my favorite Italian restaurant to experience their new happy hour take out. (Piccolo Angolo, Jane and Hudson streets in the Village). I got a nice san gria and a few freshly made pieces of garlic bread and went to a nearby little park to eat and drink. It was a nice break. Also, in the 9 block walk to Piccolo I noticed at least five other places that never have happy hours having them now. Maybe it will help them survive. These were small places so they don't have a lot of financial reserve and every little bit helps. Salute! temp today 98.3

Journal of the Plague Year, Day 55. First, the virus came for the Chinese, but I did nothing because I wasn't Chinese.

Then it came for the New Yorkers, but I did nothing because I wasn't a New Yorker.

Then it came for the nursing home residents, but I did nothing because I wasn't a nursing home resident.

Then it came for the minorities, but I did nothing because I wasn't black or Hispanic.

Then it came for the prisoners, but I did nothing because I wasn't a prisoner.

Then it came for the slaughter house workers but I did nothing because I wasn't a slaughter house worker.

Then the scientists said it would last all year, but I did nothing because the P******** said it would be over by summer.

Then the doctors said to wear a mask, but I did nothing because the P******** never wore a mask.

Now I'm alone in the ER about to be intubated. My family isn't here yet so I can't say goodbye to them before they put me under. I'm a white R*********. How could this happen to me?

Explanation: In 1946 German clergyman Martin Niemoller wrote the original version of this piece as a way of confessing his guilty behavior during the rise of the Nazis. This updating is not meant to equate the death from WWII with COVID19, at least not yet, and the voice I am using is not mine but that of a pandemic denier. If we are remembering veterans on Memorial day we should also remember what made their sacrifice necessary. What is similar in both times is denial. When you avoid facing reality, the rise of Nazis or a world wide plague, it sometimes comes back to hurt you really badly. temp today 98.3

Journal of the Plague Year, Day 56. A few weeks ago I wrote about a Starbucks in The Village opening up for take out. When coming back from work today up in Harlem, at 110th street and Lenox avenue the local poor man's Starbucks was opening. Dunking Donuts (aka Dunkin) right at the entrance of the subway at 110th street was opening for the first time since the lock down. Next door is a bodega which has been opened the entire time, but this Dunkin is going to add a little life to the corner. Across 110th street is the northern end of Central Park with lots of benches and lawns for hanging out and finishing your coffee and donuts. Racially and economically the neighborhoods are pretty different but both seem to be slowly opening with mostly, but not entirely, masked people hanging out. I just hope both places don't open up too fast since I'm not ready for a second wave of the virus just yet. temp today 98.7

Journal of the Plague Year, Day 57. Last Thursdays I had my first CORVID nasal test. It was supposed to go to the lab on Friday and return by yesterday, but it went out on Saturday and isn't back yet. Yesterday I took another CORVID test which I think was sent out. The point is that a lot of people are asking for tests but the labs that do them might be overwhelmed. And that's just talking about the numbers and logistics of the testing system and not how accurate the tests are from company to company. I hope this gets sorted out before I end up on a ventilator because of a faulty lab test. temp today 98.9

Journal of the Plague Year, Day 58. I was watching the news tonight about rioting in Minneapolis. Almost every rioter, cop, and reporter were wearing masks. Even in the middle of violence and anger people still remember that this is necessary. By contrast, a news clip of T**** signing an executive order with three of his advisors in the room had nobody with a mask. I guess they're just more health conscious in Minnesota. temp today 98.3

Journal of the Plague Year, Day 59. Everyone is trying to adapt to the quarantine. I've been told that even the porn sites are advertising that you should "Stay Home and Stay safe" by watching their porn sites. These come-ons are followed by more explicit suggestions that I need not go into. Some are even giving discounts for those who subscribe. At least, that's what I've been told. temp 98.5

Journal of the Plague Year, Day 60. Gov C**** recently signed a bill protecting nursing home owners from civil suits related to COVID and was roundly attacked since he had gotten campaign contributions from some of these people. There is a lot of corruption in politics but that doesn't mean that every decision is made on the basis of campaign donations. There are many nursing homes where owners make a fortune by providing poor services but there are also a lot of places that have done there best and simply couldn't handle the emergency. Many nursing homes and assisted livings, especially the non-profit ones, operate on thin margins and I know from my own that when the pandemic broke it was sometimes impossible to get protective equipment in adequate amounts at any price. Mary Manning Walsh, one of the best if not the best nursing home in Manhattan had more reported deaths from COVID than any other. But, if you mixed impossible situations, incomplete information, pissed off relatives, and a surplus of lawyers in New York, you could end up with a lot of lawsuits that can drive a nursing home or assisted living into bankruptcy. Over the decades many nursing homes in Manhattan have closed and that's why it's sometimes hard to get a nursing home bed in Manhattan at all. Advocates for immunity for NH and ALF owners say that gross negligence will still be prosecuted. I'm don't know if that's actually true, but I do know that even the most trivial lawsuit costs a fortune to defend against. By the way, I don't have any investment in any NH or ALF so there's no financial benefit of me protecting them, but I've worked in enough of them to know that they are not all rolling in money because of inadequate care. temp today 97.3

Journal of the Plague Year, Day 61. Sunday May 31, 2020. It would be nice if catastrophes could be spaced out with no overlap. First the epidemic, later the economic collapse and then the demonstrations and riots. That's not the way it happens. Over the last few nights large demonstrations, some of them including violence, have happened in downtown areas, though not in my particular neighborhood. By the accounts that I've read in the papers and seen on TV, and reports from friends of mine, almost all of the demonstrations were peaceful but a small number were violent, mostly against property but occasionally people. A local restaurant owner I know was worried that a curfew to restore order would force him to close much earlier and reverse some of the progress on opening that has been happening in the neighborhood. I heard that D******* is against a curfew, but since he sometimes changes his mind there's no telling what will actually happen. We'll see what happens over the next few days. temp today 98.5

Journal of the Plague Year, Day 62. I'm trying to stay on topic with the COVID pandemic, which I have some expertise in, and not get distracted with the demonstrations over the Lloyd death which I know no more about than everyone else. But there is one area they overlap. Many demos have been in Union Square about a mile from my house, but even in the far West Village there are signs of it. The local police station has one of its streets blocked off by barriers even though there are no demos in this neighborhood, and there are a few cops on that street standing guard. D******* changed his mind, as I thought he would, and announced a curfew but one starting at 11 PM. Most of the demo violence happens late. By doing it this way, at least for now, it allows more stores to stay open in spite of the COVID lock down but takes a step to controlling late night violence. I don't know if it will work, but it's a compromise that might allow both emergencies to be handled at the same time at least a little bit. We'll see if it works. Tomorrow back to COVID stuff, I hope. temp today 97.8

Journal of the Plague Year, Day 63. Lots of stores with plywood covering where their windows used to be in my neighborhood. But I promised to get back to COVID. For about 10 days all the staff at my ALF have been tested for COVID. today the results came back. Nobody tested positive of the 100 or so staffers, including myself. Not only did this indicate that the policies at the ALF were working (lots of PPE, social distancing and isolation) but that the staff was also careful when they went home or traveled outside. I don't know if we can keep this good record up, or even if it's as good as it seems given the possibility of false negative lab errors. But let's take this good news at face value for the time being. A little good news now is valuable. temp today 9.0

Journal of the Plague Year, Day 64. While COVID has taken everyone's attention because of its suddenness and lethality, the rest of medical care has to go on. When I see patients now it's usually in their room for social distancing reasons, and I have to wear gloves and face mask. Also, being away from my computer I have to remember every point I wanted when I go to them and have to remember everything they said, which is often a lot, when I come back and start writing my note. As patients and families get nervous about being out of touch with each other they make more complaints, some real and some anxiety induced, and that leads to more tests, which leads to more questions about test results and more time spent dealing with issues which aren't so critical. You end up spinning your wheels a lot, while people who don't complain and are stoic have problems which are not detected or addressed. Everything is slowed. I hope things get back to normal soon, but I worry about all the undetected illness that has been going on that will surface then. It will be busy. Maybe better news tomorrow. temp yesterday was 97.0 not 9.0. that's what happens when you do you typing at midnight. temp today, I'm pretty sure, was 97.7

Journal of the Plague Year, Day 65. Enough whining about me. Let me describe what the rest of the staff is experiencing. Most of the staff are low paid young minority women. When this started they were very worried about catching COVID since it wasn't clear just how contagious or deadly it was. They were also concerned about bringing it home to their families, a problem I don't have. But, they came in and all positions on all shifts were covered, I think. As time went on the PPE got better with surgical gowns and face shields joining the face masks and gloves we started with. Also, as a little perk, the facility started to give free lunches three days a week. This wasn't just to keep them in the building during work hours, but also to thank them for coming in and working hard. And, they're doing a good job since none of them have tested positive for the virus at our most recent testing. temp today 97.6

Journal of the Plague Year, Day 66. More grasping at straws to look for an end to the pandemic. In Greenwich Village one of the buildings of the former St. Vincent's Hospital has been taken over by Lenox Hill Hospital to form Lenox Hill Greenwich Village which is a free standing ER affiliated with, but not attached to, a hospital. When this started a large trailer truck, which looked like a refrigerator trailer, was parked outside this ER. Hospitals all over the city were doing this since their morgues were filled to capacity and they needed to hold bodies until funeral arrangements could be made. I don't know if any bodies were actually stored in the Lenox Hill site, but yesterday it was removed. It appears that maybe the overwhelming wave of deaths has peaked and hospital and ER capacity is now sufficient to handle our present level of illness. Let's hope those cases and those trailers don't come back in the future. temp today 97.4

Journal of the Plague Year, Day 67. I've been posting my temperatures each day to give a little personal touch to this story. Today after a nice long hot bath in my tub,which has a Jacuzzi built in (hot baths are good for arthritic knees and backs) I waited 10 minutes and took my temp, which was 99.4. It didn't seem right, so I took some cool diet soda, waited another ten minutes and took my temp again. 98.5. This is one of the reasons medical people don't get too upset about a degree or less variation from normal. It has to be a few degrees above normal before we really worry. At work we've been using 100.0 as the cut off that determines if a persons stays or goes home. I realize that this medical fact isn't as interesting as talking about virus mortality and looter violence but some days are just quieter than others. Tomorrow-the great experiment. temp today after a large bowl of cacio e pepe spaghetti 99.1

Journal of the Plague Year, Day 68. Sunday June 7, 2020. The great experiment in underway. What form of reopening can occur without a new spike in COVID cases? The partyers down in Florida, Texas and Georgia seemed to avoid wearing masks pretty consistently. Demonstrators in a lot of cities, including NYC seemed to mostly wear masks, from what I've seen of the videos. If you saw something different, let me know. In any case, the COVID rate for some of those states is slowly increasing. Will it level off or spike? The demonstrations are all over the country and maybe someone will be able to watch for spikes or lack of spikes and correlate with mask use. This is complicated and unclear, at least for now. But until there is treatment or a vaccine, masks and isolation are the best we have. temp today 98.3

Journal of the Plague Year, Day 69. Yesterday I walked up to my favorite Italian restaurant, Piccolo Angolo for their happy hour. Garlic bread and a few glasses of san gria. The four block walk up Hudson street was packed with people doing the same at virtually every restaurant and bar on the street. Many of them had a table or two in front where people were sitting. Many were without face masks and I wondered how people can still be so confident that they won't be touched. NY Magazine today had a brief answer. They had a few pages about the different ways people are coping and they introduced new terms: "quarantine pods" and "quarantine bubble". This is when a person has a few good friends, relatives, room mates, co-workers, etc who spend so much time together that they figure if one gets it they all get it, so they might as well relax and give in to the inevitable. Or maybe they figure they will all avoid it somehow. Good luck to each of these pods or bubbles, they may need it. temp today 95.7.

Journal of the Plague Year, Day 70. The World Health Organization came out with a statement that very few cases of COVID are spread by asymptomatic people. Almost all people spreading COVID have some warning symptoms. that hasn't been my experience. Of the 11 people who have tested positive for COVID 7 went to the ER for falls (about our average, we have a lot of falls), two for confusion or unresponsiveness, and two were detected as part of a work up for a completely unrelated matter. WHO says that maybe some of these people were presymptomatic, that is if they had been allow to avoid the ER they would have developed the typical symptoms. Maybe, but that doesn't help us when somebody has a problem right now and we have to determine if there has been an exposure to COVID immediately, not somewhere down the line. In any case, people are still being cautious no matter what WHO says. If I were more creative I could write a whole skit on WHO tells us to watch for COVID. Bud: WHO is telling us to watch out for COVID. Lou: WHO is telling us? Bud: That's right. Lou: What's right? Bud: WHO's right. Lou: That's what I'm asking, WHO's right and WHO's asking. Bud: That's right for both. Lou: Right for what? Bud: Right for WHO. Lou: WHO? Bud: Yes. Anyway, a much better, though older, version of this is on Youtube. temp today 96.5

Journal of the Plague Year, Day 71. The city is now on the third day of opening up a little. I told about people going to happy hours at the partially opened bars and restaurants. Now the rest of the city is opening up with about 400,000 people going back to work in construction and manufacturing. What I noticed is that the subways are a little more crowded. AM rush hour is about the same at 8:30 with less than a half dozen people per car. Evening rush hour is more crowded with 15-20 people per care as compared to less than ten before. Also, on some of the subway stations they have stenciled foot prints with social distancing warnings every 6 feet apart along the subway platform. I don't know how they will handle this once the rest of the city opens, but it is a small step. temp today 97.8

Journal of the Plague Year, Day 72. Maybe another sign of reopening. The ALF where I work has been on isolation. We haven't taken in any new admission, but many of our residents have gone to rehab or to permanent nursing home placement and even a few who died. Although nationally ALFs have about a 20% vacancy rate, we were always filled with a waiting list of weeks to months. This could be because we are one of the few ALFs that take Medicaid or maybe just because we're so damn good. In any case, we now have about a 15% vacancy because we haven't taken anybody in for four months. Starting soon we'll be admitting new residents. We want to fill up our beds and serve the community like we're supposed to, and people in the community need services we can provide, even if they have to risk a COVID exposure because we are a congregate facility. As much as COVID overshadows everything, there are still people with other needs that need to be met. temp today 98.4

Journal of the Plague Year, Day 73. Nursing homes have been criticized for not doing more to monitor and treat COVID cases, with terrible results. I'm not sure about all the details of what they did, as both good and bad nursing homes had bad results, but I can offer some light on this from the point of view of an assisted living facility, which I do know about. For example, the state has required that all ALF staff get tested twice a week and has supplied equipment for it. But, they aren't paying for the processing. In my facility that comes to $14,000 a week (100 staff, $70 per test twice a week) and virtually none of it is covered by any private or public insurance company. In a few months this comes to over $100,000 which is one per cent of the total operating budget of the facility. That's assuming the mandate won't continue even longer. ALF and nursing home budgets are not infinitely expandable. Some nursing homes are profitable by both good and bad methods but a lot operate on thin margins. Eventually what could happen in NYC might replicate what happened in Manhattan where there is a shortage of long term care nursing home beds. Converting a property from nursing home to luxury, or even market rate, apartments is one of the things that has led to many nursing home closings over the years. This could be worse unless funding increases or unfunded mandates decrease. temp today 97.7

Journal of the Plague Year, Day 74. Today I'm talking trash. This isn't related to COVID except maybe in the most indirect way. A week ago when demonstrations on BLM and Floyd were at there height, so was some rioting and looting. Sidewalk litter baskets were set on fire or tossed through store windows according to many media and neighborhood accounts. As a result, every litter basket in the entire neighborhood was removed. In the eight block walk from my breakfast bagel shop to home I didn't see one trash basket, on intersections where there would usually be 3 or 4. Today, I noticed that they were all back. Some were overflowing, as usual, and some were half empty, but they were all around. The streets themselves are dirty because alternate side parking is suspended and there is no street sweeping. Whether recepticals for trash will add to the cleanliness of the city and maybe cut down on infectious disease is doubtful, but at least we'll have a nicer environment in which to get sick. Tomorrow-Masks! temp today 98.4

Journal of the Plague Year, Day 75. Sunday June 14. How hard is it to wear a mask? As rules loosen up more and more people are out without masks. In the sidewalk bar/restaurant happy hours, on the streets, walking their dogs, biking, going to T**** rallies, etc, etc. Maybe they'll get lucky with open air instead of a closed room, or warm sunny weather with a nice breeze to dispense the germ laden droplets. Maybe. Or maybe they won't get lucky and the virus will take off again. I know it's uncomfortable until you get use to it. So is a ventilator. temp today 97.2

Journal of the Plague Year, Day 76. The damage to health of not wearing masks is bad enough, but a few small business owners, restaurant owners and customers I've spoken to are also worried that Phase 2 will be delayed. It would legally allow side walk dining and start to open up more stores. But if the COVID cases start going up this is all out of the question. Then the problem becomes will we go back to more restrictions, which people will hate, or put up with the eventual increase in deaths. Let's hope the winds keep blowing and the sun keeps shining to disperse those deadly little germ laden droplets and save us from ourselves. temp today 97.9

Journal of the Plague Year, Day 77. The opening of bars and restaurants in NY in phase 1 and the openings in Jersey in phase 2 are encouraging only if done correctly. Yesterday I saw a short piece on the news about Leo's Grand Vue in Hoboken which some of us on this friends list know well. It is an old school red sauce place, open for 80 years, and a virtual shrine to Frank Sinatra, who was raised in Hoboken. They briefly described how the place is opening and serving meals but only outside on the sidewalks. They always had a few tables but the news piece appeared to show a lot more tables across the street. If you go to Google maps and look up Leo's at 2nd and Grand street in Hoboken and go to the street view you see that on the corners around Leo's there are very wide sidewalks. I hope they're doing well with sidewalk tables. I'd like to go back there some time. As a matter of fact, I'm off on Monday's so I wonder if they are open for lunch. I'm assuming, given it's popularity that dinners there under phase 2, 3 or whatever will always be packed. Maybe lunch so I can get a little taste of normal life. temp today 98.1

Journal of the Plague Year, Day 78. Yesterday I wrote about how Jersey was ahead of New York since they were in phase 2 and we were still in phase 1. It looks like that might change soon. C**** says that on Monday June 22 NY can go into phase 2. D******* is being more cautious saying that there are still details to be worked out. In any case it looks like it's close. But, there are still maskless hoards of revelers around Manhattan, and who knows how many cases of COVID incubating from partying and demonstrating a few weeks ago. Let's hope the numbers stay low. We'll show Jersey who can party! temp today 98.3

Journal of the Plague Year, Day 79. Yesterday I was cautiously looking forward to phase 2 on Monday. Today a restaurant owner was complaining a lot about how it is being done. Places don't just open, they are supposed to fill out a form which will be available tomorrow. According to him 25,000 eating places in the city are supposed to fill out a form they haven't seen yet, and don't know what it asks for, by Monday. This will determine how many tables can be set outside and a lot more details. This might be chaos, and if it is remember you heard it here first. I hope we get these procedures down pat before the next pandemic hits. temp today 98.3

Journal of the Plague Year, Day 80. Just a post in favor of sentimental nostalgia. Vera Lynn, an English singer from WWII just died. She sang a sentimental song called "We'll Meet Again," which was very popular and ironically used at the end of the movie "Dr. Strangelove." Another song of the times was "Lili Marlene" popular in Germany, US, England simultaneously, and also sentimental and hopeful. Both are on Youtube. These sweet songs came out of one of the worst times in human history. Will our moderately bad time of human history produce anything similar? Beyonce's stuff is too upbeat. Maybe Taylor Swift? Where are the McGarrigle sisters when you need them? temp today 98.3

Journal of the Plague Year, Day 81. Lots of these posts I've been writing are directly related to life and death decisions we collectively are making. Here is something a little more low key. Yesterday I passed through Penn Station at about 5 PM. Normally, BC (before COVID) this place would be packed with people shoulder to shoulder. This time it was pretty well spaced out, lots of people but nothing like the usual Friday night crowd. Most with masks, some without, like the rest of the city. This was just to give a little taste of a random observation which may or may not be significant. But, the more of these little observations we can make now, maybe the more we will remember when this is over and we have to prepare for the next virus somewhere down the line. temp today 98.4

Journal of the Plague Year, Day 82, Sunday June 21. My dad and I argued over many things, including cigarettes. He thought they wouldn't hurt him in spite of 1-2 packs per day. On his virtual death bed at the Bronx Veterans Hospital, after an unsuccessful surgery for lung cancer, he looked up at me and said "was it really the smoking that did it." It almost moved me to tears. Now I see young people without masks or caution ignoring CORVID. A few interviews with young people who actually got CORVID and survived showed how they finally realized, and almost paid the ultimate price, that yes, it was the CORVID that made you sick and almost killed you. Sometimes we don't have the discipline to do what we should to be healthy, otherwise I would be 60 pounds lighter and exercise daily. But at least we need to recognize what we should try to do instead of death defying denial. temp today 97.6

Journal of the Plague Year, Day 83. Yesterday, NYC was in phase 1 isolation. today started phase 2. Since so many people were stretching phase 1 rules I didn't think there would be much change when we went to phase 2. I was probably wrong. This morning when I went out to get my morning bagel and coffee I passed 2 restaurants and a coffee shop that already had a lot of tables out on the side walk and in one of the traffic lanes on Hudson street. At 10 AM! On the news tonight they had a report from Arthur Avenue, my old neighborhood, and there were lots of restaurants with lots of tables. The city is jumping into phase 2 enthusiastically. Tomorrow, weather permitting, I'll be sitting at one of these sidewalk tables for dinner. More details to follow. temp today is 98.3

Journal of the Plague Year, Day 84. First day of phase 2 and the restaurants are starting to open. I was the first one at Piccolo Angolo eating al fresco early at 5:30. Walking around the neighborhood most restaurants were open and few were completely filled, at least not that early. The real test will come on the weekend. Dinners Friday, Saturday, and Sunday and brunches Saturday and Sunday are the normal heavy times. If the weather is good they should be packed. This isn't the most startling or significant news, considering how the city is slowly recovering in terms of actual deaths (reportedly less than 10 a day), but it's the one thing I can report that I saw myself. temp today 98.1

Journal of the Plague Year, Day 85. Things at work eased up a tiny bit. Under the direction of the NY State Department of Health, all staff were tested for CORVID twice a week. This week the DOH said we could test once a week instead. It still costs a lot of money and still annoying but no clearly positive cases. One problem has been with a false positive. A staff member had a negative, a positive, and two negative tests all taken within a few days of each other. All came back together and the most likely explanation is that the positive test was a lab error, a false positive. This is one of the reasons lots of government agencies and individual institutions and doctors, including me, don't like ordering tests unless they are absolutely unavoidable. This person could have been put on isolation for two weeks which would stress him and the facility which has staff stretched a little thin. Tomorrow, false negatives. temp today 98.9

Journal of the Plague Year, Day 86. Yesterday, false positives. Today, false negatives. These are tests that are incorrect because they say a person is negative for a disease, like COVID, but the person actually has it. The test wasn't sensitive or accurate enough to detect it. The problem with a contagious disease with a false negative is that the person thinks he is not infectious and can't make others sick, when he actually can. If this person follows all the rules, masks/distance, there will be less contagion, but nobody with a false negative is going to self-isolate for two weeks, which would be the proper procedure if possible. The false positives and negatives, and the newness of the tests being used, is one of the reasons the DOH has been hesitant to allow widespread testing in nursing homes and assisted living facilities, where overconfidence involving an inaccurate tests can have a really bad result. As the tests get more reliable, and the total numbers go down, and the staff and facility is able to isolate patients these rules may loosen up. But not yet. temp today 98.3

Journal of the Plague Year, Day 87. I could write a negative post about how Florida and Texas have to close bars because they killed people by ignoring warnings. But, I'll write something upbeat instead. The assisted living where I work has been on isolation, and one of the policies has been to not take in new residents. Next week this changes. We usually are completely filled with a waiting list of a dozen or so people. Now we have 20 empty apartments out of 127 because of deaths and transfers to nursing homes. This is over 3 months and is much higher than our usual turnover. Next we have new people moving in, maybe 3 or 4. It will take a few months to fill up completely, but this is a good start. Virus or no virus, many people still need the services of an ALF and that's just what we're here for. temp today 98.2

Journal of the Plague Year, Day 88. I avoided this yesterday, but on a Saturday night, bar behavior becomes important. Florida and Texas aren't closing down everything, just bars. Of all the indoor activity, bars are probably the most dangerous with COVID (and maybe other times also). People are face to face, masks down to drink, talking, laughing, whatever, maybe for hours. Church services are briefer and people aren't talking much, from what I remember. Restaurants space people out with tables and seats. But, there's no spacing in bars. I hope these young folks survive, or at least learn a little caution if they get sick and survive. temp today. 97.9

Journal of the Plague Year, Day 89, Sunday June 28. Gay Pride Day. Usually there is a big parade with the post parade partiers congregating in the bars and restaurants of the West Village and Chelsea afterwards. Today there was not big parade, but an official parade or maybe 1-2 thousand on the West Side and Fifth Avenue. But, the bars along Hudson were packed, maybe with Pride celebrators maybe with random partyers. The area around Stonewall was packed with demostrators, partiers, and several closed off streets. It wasn't as extravagant as the usual Pride weekends, but it wasn't a normal Sunday afternoon either. The fiftieth Pride celebration was supposed to be special but I didn't think people thought it would be special in quit this way. temp today 98.6

Journal of the Plague Year, Day 90. I signed my Will today. I should have done this a long time ago when it wouldn't have been under so dramatic circumstances. I'm very good at procrastinating, which is why this has been put off so long. But, even I have a limit and eventually have to get things done. I don't know what will be left of my estate. I'm hoping to use up my retirement accounts to live on. My apartment is valuable but I can't predict if I'll be living in it until the end, or if I'll end up in an ALF or nursing home. Don't want to get too morbid about this, but making out a Will tends to bring out the dark side under the best of circumstances, even though I'm ok at this exact moment. temp today 98.1

Journal of the Plague Year, Day 91. I hate updates. Just as I was getting used to FB they decide to change the format. I'm minimally literate in computer stuff so change like this throws me. The update said I could go back to the "classic" format but I couldn't figure out how to do that either. Anyway, back to COVID related stuff. Sunday I got my first haircut in about four months. Astor Haircutters is a place I've gone to since I moved down to Manhattan in 1993. They're fast with a large bunch of barbers and I almost never have to wait. At 4 PM I walker in the door. They immediately took my temperature via my forehead. The guy at front who assigned me to a cutter was behind a plastic partition. Another guy took my phone number, I don't know why, maybe it was for tracing just in case, maybe it was a health department rule. The chairs are usually well separated, but they now had plastic curtains between them also. I had to wear my usual mask and the barber had on a mask and gloves. The haircut was fast and good, as usual. The cashier was also behind a plastic shield. The price went up from $18 5 months ago to $23, but since they haven't changed their prices and they obviously had new expenditures I didn't mind. Also, I think $23 is still cheap for NYC. OK, not the most dramatic sign of the times, but to give a complete picture of life in the time of CORVID I thought I would put in everything. temp today 97.9

Journal of the Plague Year, Day 92. Monday July the 6th was going to be the day that New York City went into phase 3 with indoor dining. But outside dining only started a little over a week ago and this Fourth of July weekend could easily bring out lots of crowds spilling out and mixing unsafely. Phase three on Monday seemed too soon. Even three friends of mine who are restaurant owners thought it was too soon. They thought that if early opening brought about another wave of infections then we would have to go back to phase one and would lose all the progress we've made over the last few months. Fortunately, the state, or whoever makes decisions in the state, realized this and they cancelled the phase 3 opening on Monday the 6th. It seems that the safest thing would be to wait 2-3 weeks after the July 4th holiday and festivities which would not only include restaurants and bars, but lots of unofficial bbq parties and who knows how much unsafe mixing. Waiting until the end of July to see if there is another spike in cases is the safest. I just hope the bars and restaurants I know can hold on that long. temp today 98.0

Journal of the Plague Year, Day 93. Walking around the West Village where there are lots of bars and restaurants, I've noticed two different reactions to the lock down. Some of these places have just closed and are waiting for phase 3 or 4, or they have just closed, like Aria on Perry Street. Others have taken an aggressive approach. Many places have put tables on the sidewalks and streets. But some of the streets have uneven surfaces, like the cute cobble stone streets of the West Village. Restaurants and bars on those streets have started to build platforms of plywood that provide flat surfaces for additional outside tables. At least a half dozen restaurants in just a four block stretch of Hudson and Perry streets have these platforms. Some places, like Cafe Dante on Perry and Hudson have just opened up in the face of COVID. In the next few months, especially as we go into phases 3 and 4, we will see which approach is correct. I hope they all survive. temp today 98.9

Journal of the Plague Year, Day 94. There's something about the re-opening that I noticed. Last Sunday, coming back from Little Italy, I had a hard time getting a cab. Very few were on the streets. When I asked the driver about it he said that the drivers are willing to work, especially when they're protected by a partition and can keep their windows open. But the customers aren't there. The small bodega around the corner from my house had reopened but only Monday to Saturday. That's when the local construction workers, their main customers, are around. No construction on Sunday, no open bodega. Whenever we do get to phase three and in door dining is allowed, will the customers come in sufficient numbers or be scared off by persist and justified COVID fears? Can indoor dining with 6 feet between tables be economically viable? I'll let you know when it happens. temp today 99.2

Journal of the Plague Year, Day 95. I've written about the opening of sidewalk bars and restaurants and the crowds of people, many maskless, who crowd around. In Westview news, a neighborhood paper in Greenwich Village, one of the owners of the White House Tavern wrote an article about this. The White Horse is a landmarked establishment opened in 1880. Dylan Thomas the poet performed his poetry there and probably drank himself to death there also. It's very historic. It's also very crowded even with just partial sidewalk business. Eytan Sugarman, one of the owners, talked about how he can't really control the crowds. He tells people to distance, wear masks, and even gives them out but people don't comply, and he can't force them to. He can always cut them off and not serve but he says that the White Horse is on the verge of closing due to finances. If true, this would be a real shame. And, he can't be the only owner in NYC with the same problem. A post on FB listed another half dozen places just in this neighborhood that are recently closing. Some will survive, but there will be a lot of damage. temp today 98.3

Journal of the Plague Year, Day 96, Sunday July 5. Last Sunday, after my haircut. I took a bar hopping tour of lower Manhattan. First to Cafe Katja on Orchard street. Inexpensive Austrian food and very good beer for a Vienner Schnitzel and dark Dunkel beer and a schnapps. They have been in business for 12 years and have won awards for best family friendly restaurant and best restaurant on the entire lower East side (where there are a thousand places to eat). But even with that, if they don't work out a deal with their landlord on rent they may have to close. What a shame. Then to Cafe Palermo for an espresso, Sambuca, and sfiogliatelle. Then to Piccolo Angolo for a happy hour san gria (ok, maybe two san grias). Then, when walking home, I saw a friend outside The Left Bank on Perry Street and stopped for another glass of wine. Fortunately, it is within staggering distance of my apartment and so I actually made it home. A good way to spend a Sunday afternoon, even with so much of the city locked down. temp today. 98.3

Journal of the Plague Year, Day 97. Yesterday I took a walk along the Hudson River in the Hudson River Park. I then walked across Canal street to Orchard street to have dinner at Cafe Katja again (see yesterdays post). I made a few observations like my previous ones and one new one. The number of people wearing masks, and wearing them correctly (wearing them under the chin doesn't count as wearing it) was roughly 50%. But, when I walked through Chinatown it seemed to me that people who appeared Asian had a much higher per cent of mask wearers. this was true throughout Chinatown except for one park at the South end of Sara Roosevelt park where lots of guys who appeared to be gambling or just playing cards, dominoes, mah jong, there appeared to be about 50% without masks. Men! These were all random observations so maybe anyone else who knows the neighborhood or what is going on down there can let me know if my observation was accurate or not. temp today. 97.7

Journal of the Plague Year, Day 98. When this pandemic started and all the ERs in NYC were packed with people and many of them with COVID there was an indirect effect on everyone else in the city who didn't have COVID. Many patients of mine who would have usually gone to the local ER refused because they thought, probably accurately, that there was a good chance they would get COVID. Now things are quieter. There are less COVID patients in the city, in the local ERs and local hospitals. Also, many of our patients who had to go to the ER, such as those who fell and hit their heads, came back to the ALF without getting COVID, at least as far as we know. This is starting the change medicine in NYC as hospitals are playing catch up. temp today. 98.5

Journal of the Plague Year, Day 99. Yesterday I mentioned how patients are behaving about medical appointments and ER visits. Now, for the doctors. On TV I'm seen some commercials by doctors or hospitals telling patients to take care of themselves and come and take care of their other medical problems. They mention that there are fewer COVID cases to reassure patients. But doctors availability is variable. We make appointments for our patients to go to a variety of doctors whose offices are outside the facility. Some are open completely, in person, just like before. Some are opened virtually and the patient is only seen remotely from a doctor at a remote location, with maybe a nurse in the actual office. Some are completely closed, especially since lots of doctors and especially mental health professionals, take vacation time in July and especially at the end of August. After Labor Day we will see if things are really back to normal, assuming no new wave of COVID. That new wave might not come until flu season later in the fall. temp today. 98.2

Journal of the Plague Year, Day 100. On day 95 I wrote about the historic White Horse tavern and how they had trouble keeping their customers distant. One of the owners even wrote an article in the local paper about how tough it was. The state had a simple solution to this problem. It pulled their liquor license. The White Horse, historic or not, is completely closed. News of this has spread through the neighborhood and all the other bars and restaurants know about it. I also saw an inspector from the NYC Buildings Department inspecting another restaurant nearby. Borough President G*** B***** speaking to our political club tonight said that the NYC Dept of Health would actually be inspecting, and maybe closing, some of these places. As a bar/restaurant lover, I feel bad about this. But, as a doctor I'm really glad they're doing this. Enjoying the night life is one thing, killing people, even accidentally, is something else entirely. temp today 97.8

Journal of the Plague Year, Day 101. Lots of Southern states are having increased hospitalizations and ICU needs. Many ICUs are almost filled and people are worried about this new situation. But, this isn't new. When I was a medical resident years ago at Overlook Hospital we had ICU beds that we always had to negotiate for. Most of our patients had private doctors and those doctors wanted the patients in the ICU as often as possible since that would give the patients more coverage and sometimes mean less work for the doctors since there would be house staff (interns and residents) who would do a lot of the work and take a lot of the late night calls. There were always borderline cases who were the sickest of the patients on the general wards, or the healthiest of the patients in the ICU, and there was always jockeying for who went where. Triage always occurred. Did the last bed in the ICU go to the old very sick person from the nursing home who you might or might not be able to save, and maybe get them another year of life, or did it go to the young person, with a family and kids, whose recovery could give them decades of life? There was always triage. As ICUs in the country now fill up with COVID patients these decisions will be made every day in every hospital. And they won't be easy decisions. temp today 98.5

Journal of the Plague Year, Day 102 (a little late). There's lots of talk about opening schools, at least partially, and what risk there is for kids and those around them. Besides COVID, there's another reason to be careful. It's always been known that schools are an incubator for contagious respiratory disease. Kids give them to each other and then it goes back to everyone's home to infect siblings, parents, grandparents. I remember a study looking at medical students who were doing a rotation in pediatrics. When they looked at how often they went to the medical school's student health clinic they found that those rotating through pediatrics had a significantly higher rate of colds and respiratory symptoms than students doing other rotations. Historically, kids and schools are major vectors for disease. I hope we dodge it this time as the schools open. Much higher stakes. temp today 98.7

Journal of the Plague Year, Day 103, Sunday July 12. I'm very worried. Today I took my usual Sunday stroll and passed through several neighborhoods in lower Manhattan. Lots of places had sidewalk tables with take out drinks and food. Hudson street and Ochard street from Kenmare to Grand were packed, standing room only. Little Italy and Bleecker from LaGuardia Place to Grove street were busy, but good spacing. But almost nobody was wearing masks on any of these streets. Young healthy beautiful people who could easily be turned into sick and dying people if things go wrong. The Times had an article about how Corpus Christi Texas, also filled with young healthy people a while back, playing in the sunny fresh sea side breezes were confident they were ok. Now they have a major crisis there. I don't know what's going to happen in NYC, but I'm very worried. temp today 98.5

Journal of the Plague Year, Day 104. Yesterday I wrote that increased people crowding together outside was dangerous and I don't know what's going to happen. Actually, I do know what's going to happen but I don't know when or how severe it will be. C**** thinks there will be a second wave of virus infections when we go to the indoor dining part of phase 3. It might be sooner. If the outdoor activities of the last few weeks are as bad as I thought, we could have a second wave of infections in a month. what we don't know if the effect of this wave. how many new cases will there be and how many new deaths. we can have more cases but fewer deaths if the cases are small in number or in healthy populations (young adults and kids) and if we continue to treat COVID more successfully. And, of course, there is always the wave that will probably come during the flu season. But, on an optimistic note, we are getting better with treatment. More on that later in the week. temp today 97.9

Journal of the Plague Year, Day 105. When this all started, my cousin Bonnie, who is in this Friends group, sent me a video of a doctor in Brooklyn who thought that the way we use ventilators in COVID patients is wrong. Standard procedures are actually making the patients sicker, he said. There is so much bad information on the internet, and so many unknown people who have made some great discovery that will reshape the world, and they want to share it. I told Bonnie that I would wait until I saw it in medical journals. I didn't have long to wait. Doctors and scientists were getting their COVID research published very quickly and stuff started to come out that COVID was not reacting the way most viruses do when a person is intubated and on a ventilator. For a variety of reasons, ventilators don't have to be the only way to get oxygen into the lungs for these patients. Now, high pressure face masks can deliver oxygen well in a lot of people. And this is only the first few months. We'll get even better with time. Thanks Bonnie. temp today. 98.5

Journal of the Plague Year, Day 106. Maybe some temporary good news. COVID infections in the South are taking off but death rates aren't. Part of this is because younger healthier people are the ones getting infected. Also, treatments are getting better. Medications like Remdisovir, steroids, blood thinners are all showing a little benefit for selected populations of patients. Not hydroxychloroquin, which might increase your chance of dying. But, the bad numbers might swamp the improved methods. If treatment improves 50% over several months, but new cases increase 100%

every week, eventually the death rate will go up and shortages of protective equipment, hospital beds, and staff time will happen all over the country. The head of the CDC said that if everyone in the country were to wear a mask the epidemic could be almost gone in about a month or two. It's sad that we have a way to stop this, but we just won't do it. temp today 98.8

Journal of the Plague Year, Day 107. A few days ago I wrote about how I was worried that a second wave would be coming because people, especially you bar/restaurant goers, were not being careful about social distancing and masks. I didn't realize that "would be coming" might be the wrong tense. It might already be hear. In the NY Daily News (which everyone should read to know what's going on in NYC) editorial they mention that the second wave is already starting. They said that the NYC health officials announced that the infection rate of COVID for 20-29 years olds increased 43% from mid to late June. A 43% increase in just two weeks is very bad, even if it only hits one small population group. This could easily spread to their other friends, parents/grandparents, co-workers, or other young people. Also, as I mentioned a few days ago, an increase in cases won't increase deaths, at least not immediately. But, maybe eventually. temp today 98.1

Journal of the Plague Year, Day 108. A few days ago the state sent out guidelines to allow visitors to adult facilities like nursing homes and ALFs. this sounded like a great thing until the Nicole, CEO at our place, sent me the actual memo and the details. The facility has to have no COVID positive tests, among residents or staff, for 28 days, sufficient staff to monitor visitors, although only 2 visitors are allowed for each resident and even then they must be spaced out. there are several pages of similar details. right now, only 10% of the adult facilities in NY State meet all the requirements and can have visitors. my place is working on it and we hope to get visitors soon. But not yet. temp today 98.8

Journal of the Plague Year, Day 109. (On day 107 I wrote "hear" instead of "here". That's what happens when you write these things in the middle of the night.). Anyway, two new terms in our vocabulary: Quarantine Pod and Quarantine Bubble. They both refer to the phenomenon of people out in public with a few good friends or relatives, none of whom are wearing masks. The idea is that they spend so much time together that if one gets infected they will all be infected anyway. But, these pods/bubbles also exist in the numerous sidewalk tables and restaurants. Even if your pod/bubble is safe, can you be sure about the ones that are just a few feet from you? And, if you're there for an hour or two eating and drinking can you be sure nothing wafts over from the other tables to infect you. As I see more places opening up I get more paranoid about safety. As I said before, the second wave may have already started. temp today 98.9

Journal of the Plague Year, Day 110 Sunday July 19th. Last week I mention how I went over to Orchard Street to have dinner and saw a lot of young people without masks or social distancing. What I didn't say was that it actually made me tearful to see it. I'm normally not over emotional, and not depressed or stressed. My job, 9-5 4 days a week is very manageable. But looking at these young folks and thinking what might come next almost brought me to tears. A few days later stats came out saying that young people 20-29 had a 43% increase in cases over the last two weeks in June confirmed my fears. Today, on Orchard street, everything calmed down. there were no crowds milling about, either maskless or shoulder to shoulder, so that was good. all the people at sidewalk table were well separated from each other, so that was good. let's hope today's facts on the street are more of a prediction of the future than last weeks. temp today 98.8

Journal of the Plague Year, Day 111. Yesterday I mentioned how I was briefly effected when I saw crowds of young people without masks. TV news showed more of this tonight with massive parties in Astoria and Long Beach. But the real stress on doctors and nurses isn't seeing foolish behavior on TV, it's in the day to day work they do in the hospitals and nursing homes. That is were stress really occurs. The suicide of ER doc Lorna Breen was in the news briefly, but what of all the others who are working silently and getting stressed? In extreme cases this can lead to burn out, depression or, worse of all, diseases of despair. This is when anyone, even random citizens, get so hopeless about life that they see no future. This results in alcoholism, drug abuse, and suicide, the three markers of diseases of despair. I don't know if this has effected the medical community. When we are through the worst of this pandemic, I hope some researcher looks back and studies what this did to the medical and nursing communities. We'll be studying how to prepare for the next epidemic with planning, vaccines, public health, sufficient supplies of PPEs, etc, but we should also study how events like this grind down the human resources too. OK, enough pessimism. Tomorrow a little lighter subject as we sloooowly move into Phase 4. temp today 98.1

Journal of the Plague Year, Day 112. As the city slowly opens up as it goes into Phase 4, there is still some work to be done on Phase 3. Specifically, restaurants are still not open for inside dining. Lots of tables are just outside on the sidewalk and traffic lanes, but not inside. The crowds that gather outside the bars and restaurants sometimes get out of control. I wrote about how the White Horse tavern lost its liquor licence for now. The other places took notice. On the same block as the White Horse is Cafe Dante. The original one has been in the Village since 1915, one of the old time Italian cafes. They built a new branch on Hudson street and it was about to open when COVID hit. It was closed before it was opened. About 2-3 weeks ago it actually did open with side walk tables. Business was good, too good. The crowds started to get big. I noticed last Saturday night that it was closed. A friend heard that the place intentionally closed on its busiest night so as not to risk losing its liquor licence. Better to lose one night's business than a liquor licence. So, with scattered bars around the city starting to get closed, there are others like Cafe Dante that are trying to be more careful.

Good luck to them. Let's hope they survive when the full reopening comes. temp today 98.2

Journal of the Plague Year, Day 113. I think the ballet has returned to NYC. Not the fancy ones in Lincoln Center, but the ballets that happen on our streets on Mondays and Thursdays or Tuesdays and Fridays early in the morning. It is the ballet of car owners trying to get a legal spot within alternate parking rules. When walking to work one morning, I saw lots of people sitting in their cars in the West Village in what looks like the old routine. They wait on the safe side of the street for the sweeper to come and clean the other empty side. Then they quickly scoot over to the empty side and sit there in their cars. They have to sit until the spot becomes legal or a traffic agent could give them a big ticket. So they sit, wait while watching the time and leave as soon as the alternate side time limit is reached. It is like a ballet of cars and drivers with minute by minute choreography until the street is safe. And then, a few days later, they do it again. These rules were suspended initially because of COVID but now it looks like it's starting to come back a little at a time. I'm so glad I got rid of my car years ago. temp today 98.4

Journal of the Plague Year, Day 114. As we slowly move into Phase 4, maybe there's a little more good news and a few more options for normal behavior. Museums and malls remain closed but many parks, the Bronx Zoo and Botanical Gardens are opened. You need reservations so that there won't be over crowding and there is plenty of room in both places, plenty to see, and can make for a pleasant day. Next to the Zoo is the Arthur Avenue neighborhood where I grew up. I haven't been up there since quarantine started but I've seen in the papers and TV, and heard from friends, that there are plenty of places there to enjoy its most important attribute: food. Plenty of restaurants, probably with plenty of sidewalk tables, cafes, specialty food stores, pastry shops, bread stores and maybe even the indoor market if it's open. A pleasant afternoon in the Zoo or

Gardens, a determined hunt for parking around Arthur Avenue, and an over-indulgence in food and drink could make for an enjoyable respite from the grueling days of quarantine. If you get up there before I do, have a drink for me. temp today 98.6

Journal of the Plague Year, Day 115. The recovery from COVID quarantines and chaos is slowly occurring. At the assisted living facility where I work there have been big changes. Before COVID all of our 127 rooms were taken and we had a long waiting list. This was at a time when ALFs nationally had an average of 20% or so vacancies. During the quarantine, we had a few deaths, many permanent transfers to nursing homes and no new people moving in. It was too dangerous to take in untested people into a facility where everyone is old and almost everyone has significant medical problems. We ended up with about 20 empty rooms. Now, that is slowly turning around. In the last few weeks we took in 3 new residents, and in the next few weeks there will be about 5 more. Needs for assisted living services out weigh possible COVID fears. The new residents all have to have negative tests, I believe, before they move in. At this rate, it will take us quite a few months to get back up to our previous level. But, at least we are starting to move in the right direction and fulfilling our mission of serving the community, which is why our facility exists in the first place. temp today 98.4

Journal of the Plague Year, Day 116. I mentioned recently that the state is allowing people to visit long relatives in long term care facilities, but there are a lot of regulations and conditions. One came into focus this week. All residents must be offered the COVID test, even if they decline it. So far about half of the residents at my facility have opted to get the test. If positive, the person will have to be on isolation for two weeks. Also, it resets the clock on when visitors could come in. The facility must be COVID clear 100% with not a single positive test. If one resident, even if asymptomatic, tests positive we will have to wait for at least 28 days before we can be open to visitors. Meanwhile, family members are coming and getting their relatives to go out for medical visits so there is some person to person contact, just not inside the facility. The nature of the test is still to be determined and will be described shortly. tempt today. 97.6

Journal of the Plague Year, Day 117, Sunday July 26. In an effort to find some signs of the city coming back to normal, I detected one more small piece of evidence. When coming back from Mulberry street and pastry at Cafe Palermo, I managed to get a taxi after walking about a block. This is the best result since this started although it could just be a piece of good luck. After giving the driver my destination, and him telling me to put my mask back on, I asked him if business was picking up. He said yes, there were more people around and the downtown part of the city was busy, but midtown was completely empty. The Times had a piece either today or yesterday about how the bustling area around the Time Life building has now turned into a ghost town. Taxi drivers are a good source of info. I guess on neighborhood at a time is the best we can do right now. temp today 97.8

Journal of the Plague Year, Day 118. There has been a lot of talk about how our response to COVID is now the "new normal". The deli worker who gave me my bec sandwich and coffee said how they are all getting used to things as they are. Their family run place is open 24-7 with the whole family pitching in. I started to think about what will happen when we try to get back to the "old" normal. Which of our emergency actions will be continued. A piece of legislation has been introduced into the NYC Council to allow the side walk and street tables and platforms to continue even if indoor dining resumes. Several good reasons. Indoor dining might still require social distancing to prevent virus spread and so business might not really be back to normal even in Phase 4. Also, as long as the weather holds out, outdoor dining is kind of pleasant. Not when it's raining or the temp is 95 but at other times. I hope they keep some of these new policies even as we do progress into Phase 4. temp today 98.3

Journal of the Plague Year, Day 119. Getting back to anything like normal will involve getting kids back in school. As previously mentioned, these kids were vectors for respiratory disease spreading even before COVID. Now there will be a million of them walking around and going to school. but what kind of school? Other members of my political club who are deeply involved in educational issues say that the guidelines for reopening the schools are chaotic. Even within the NYC school system there are variations in school size, budgets, enrollment, staffing and probably other problems we haven't even discovered yet. And we don't have much time unless the opening date is pushed back, which might happen. I don't have any kids of my own to worry about, but the staff at my ALF has a lot of young workers who do have kids. The residents have lots of grandkids who they might see when they go outside the building. It only takes one infected kid to indirectly and accidentally send the virus into the facility. And lots of people will have intense opinions about this. I'm glad I only have to take care of people's medical problems and can leave this potential mess to others. temp today. 98.3

Journal of the Plague Year, Day 120. Cars. Yes, cars. When this all started in March, people who didn't want to take the still risky subways started driving into Manhattan for whatever work was open. Commuting time increased a lot and finding street parking also increased. With time more people started taking the subway and driving got easier. but now lots of restaurants, at least in The Village are setting up tables in the street and on the sidewalks and also the street lane closest to the sidewalk. Lots of parking spots have disappeared but we know from conflicts over the Citibike bicycle placement that neighborhoods fight for their parking spots. In July and August many people leave the city even before COVID. When I had a car years ago, July and August were the easiest time for parking. I always got a spot within a block of my apartment. After Labor Day this year, these expatriots from vacations will come back and be fighting for spots with the many space taking restaurant tables. If you see reports in the papers and on TV, remember you heard it here first. temp today 98.1

Journal of the Plague Year, Day 121. Cars too. Although some are trying to make NYC a bicycle city instead of a car city, there are still a lot of things going on with our gas guzzling devices. NY Daily News had an article today about yellow Taxis and a 90% drop in trips since the quarantine started. An op-ed piece by the TLC head said that some yellow cabs and some for hire drivers were making as much now as before. I think that is a small minority. They are kept afloat because the city is paying $53 a ride for them to deliver needed food and medicine, although $53 is a lot more than I tip when I get a delivery. My doorman who drove in from Queens took 45 minutes before quarantine and 1.5 hours during it since lots of people didn't want to take the subway. It also took him about an hour to find a parking spot in the West Village instead of the usual 10-15 minutes. Now he uses the subways. And remember, there will be a lot of fighting for parking after Labor Day when local car owners who are returning from vacation, commuters driving in, and restaurant/bar owns who want that curbside space will all be fighting for parking spots at the same time. There are only so many spaces. Good luck to them, I'll stick to the subways while spacing and masking as much as possible. temp today 98.3

Journal of the Plague Year, Day 122. When I heard that Herman Cain died I was surprised that I felt really bad about it. Of course, when he was running for president I didn't agree with him on any issue whatsoever, except possibly for a common love of pizza. But it just seemed that this is another example of someone causing his own death, whether he picked up the bug at the T**** rally or anyplace else where he was walking around without a mask. Ignorance, stubbornness, desire to kiss up to T**** or whatever, should not result in the death penalty. Like the young people on Orchard street I described a few weeks ago, or my own patients who "don't like pills" and let their deadly diseases go untreated until they die from preventable conditions, seeing someone die from non-compliance is just a sad thing. Since there are other politicians who brag about their avoidance of masks, there will be more deaths like this among political leaders and those around them. Sad. temp today 98.4

Journal of the Plague Year, Day 123. I just read my cousin Bonnie's post about how everyone at Menlo Mall was wearing masks. But when I went out and saw people sitting on sidewalk tables almost nobody had masks. so, what accounts for the difference. Maybe it's NY vs NJ rules and regs, maybe it's Boomers vs Millenials, but I think it's more likely Indoors vs Outdoors. In a mall where everyone is breathing the same air, what exactly are you breathing? Is the air being recirculated, filtered, fresh air from outside, or what? does the sunny breezy outdoor environment really sterilize those toxic little droplets that drift from table to table? Who knows? Maybe the Outdoor people are right and the increased cases seen a few weeks ago will not translate into more clinical disease and death. Maybe they're wrong. After this is over, I hope some epidemiologist figures out what really helps and what really doesn't so maybe we'll be ready for the second wave of COVID or the first wave of whatever comes next out of China, Mexico, or the Middle East. temp today 98.3

Journal of the Plague Year, Day 124. Sunday August 2. Lots of information is coming out about COVID. Some seems accurate and some contradictory. A single research study on kids says younger than 10 has a low level of transmission and infection, but 11-19 both are close to adult levels. Another study says kids less than 10 are loaded with COVID particles but not infectious. What to make of it? Most medical research takes years to do and years to get published. For COVID, these studies are being done in a few months and published just as quickly. In general, be skeptical about any new breakthroughs or projections unless they are reproduced several times. The only real agreement is always wear masks and social distance. That's still good advice. temp today 97.6

Journal of the Plague Year, Day 125. I've been trying to get together with some others, but I'm worried about healthy people being carriers. If a person gets COVID and recovers all the symptoms might be gone but there still might be carrying the virus in their noses and throats. We see this is other diseases like MRSA and c. diff where people can have t various bugs, and be able to spread them, but have no symptoms themselves. With COVID we know that there are some people who are completely without symptoms but have viruses that they can spread, and possibly even if they have been infected and now are personally protected by antibodies. I hope we can figure this out, otherwise I'll be paranoid about getting close to anyone anytime. temp today 96.9

Journal of the Plague Year, Day 126. The issue of wearing masks and how that infringes on our constitutional right to spread disease and kill people, including ourselves, has been compared to many other infringements. We are obligated to wear seat belts, can't smoke in restaurants and bars, no shoes no service or no pants no service in restaurants and bars, even some beachfront ones, wear masks during flu season if not innoculated and working in health care facilitites, vaccinations before going to public schools, not carrying loaded guns on airplanes, and countless others. You can add in your favorite if you want to help me beat this issue to death. We are going to see so many more maskless people get sick and die, but I just hope they don't take too many careful people with them. tempt today 97.8

Journal of the Plague Year, Day 127. My state Senator B*** H****** had a Face Book post where he showed himself getting injected with an experimental COVID vaccine. I didn't know vaccine testing was so far along in NYC but apparently it is. He also mentioned a website where you can go to register as a volunteer in future vaccine tests: coronavirus-preventionnetwork.org. I went there and registered even though I never heard of this before. I hope that B*** screened them carefully. They seem ok. they don't advocate any one test site or program and they seem to be a clearing house for many different national programs. I registered with some simple information (they didn't ask for social security number or credit card number or anything really sensitive) and I'm now waiting to hear from any program. when I get specifics I'll decide to participate if they seem reasonable and well planned. temp today 97.5

Journal of the Plague Year, Day 128 (a little late). Yesterday, the Department of Health (the DOH) swooped into my alf to test the residents for COVID. One of the requirements for long term care facilities to reopen for visitors was that all the residents should be offered COVID testing. At my place about half the residents requested it. For a change, instead of just mandating it, the DOH actually did the testing, which I think relieves the facility of the cost. Seven DOH nurses came early in the morning and set up camp in one of the meeting rooms. It almost looked like a surgical suite with every space filled with equipment, paperwork, and material for the tests. They went through the building and tested all though who wanted it and hadn't changed their minds. When I asked one of the nurses when the results would be back, she didn't know. None of us know, but we're hoping asap. If any of the tests are positive we will have to do some contact tracing ourselves and we'll have to be on isolation for another 28 days. We're waiting and hoping. temp today 98.0

Journal of the Plague Year, Day 129. A topic that has come up recently has been a criticism of C**** for ordering nursing homes to take COVID patients back from hospitals. C**** has said that the spike in NH deaths occurred before the return of these patients because of infections brought in by staff. I don't have all these stats in front of me so I'll give him the benefit of the doubt. But another point that nobody has made is that sending patients to NH may have been the only option. There were two choices. Keep them in the hospitals or send them to Rehab/NH. At that time the hospitals were swamped and barely keeping up with new patients. The nursing homes were risky but safer than the hospitals. We didn't have an unlimited number of choices. If the patients had been isolated at the NH it would have been safer than the overwhelmed hospitals. Unfortunately, many NH, even the best, couldn't isolate patients. But hospitals appeared to be as much a real death sentence as the nursing homes later turned out to be. temp today 97.4

NOTE; I'LL BE TAKING THE WEEKENDS OFF FROM POSTING. TIME ISN'T A FACTOR, BUT GETTING NEW INFORMATION FROM MY POINT OF VIEW IS. LOTS OF STUFF ON COVID IS COMING OUT IN THE PRESS, BUT FOR THAT YOU CAN READ THE PAPERS (SOME PEOPLE ACTUALLY DO STILL READ PAPERS), OR WATCH TV NEWS. I'M TRYING TO REPORT THINGS FROM THE TRENCHES THAT DON'T APPEAR ANYPLACE ELSE. I'LL STILL NUMBER THE DAYS I DON'T WRITE, JUST NO POSTS, AT LEAST FOR NOW.

Journal of the Plague Year, Day 32. This doesn't relate to COVID only, but to medical care in general. You may have noticed this if you watch all the interviews on TV with doctors and nurses during the COVID pandemic. A significant proportion of health care providers are foreign born. 25-30% of doctors and about 15% of nurses are foreign born. Most who come to the US become citizens, but not all. Some parts of the country depend more heavily on foreign born. Some areas of health care are more dependent also. It's hard to go into a nursing home in the NYC are without seeing the high percent of nurses from the Philippines or the Caribbean. Home health aides are the same. Geriatrics, my field, also has a high per cent of foreign born. Recently, there have been proposals to make it harder for legal immigrants to come into the US. If this happens, expect health care, especially in some areas and some specialties. temp today 98.2

Journal of the Plague Year, Day 133 (last post should not have been day 32, but 132. oops). One of the things I like about posting is that now and then I discuss something that the main stream media hasn't picked up on. I like to scoop the NY Times whenever possible.

On day 121 I posted about the fight over parking spots. Car owners, restaurant owners and bikers all want those lanes available for parking, eating or biking. Today the Times had an article entitled "Turn lane, bike lane, or cafe? The struggle grows." They describe a lot of the conflict that I predicted, except that I thought it would happen after Labor Day when the car driving vacationers return. Maybe the fight has already started, according to the Times. We'll see. I didn't see the authors of the article, Winnie Hu and Nate Schweber, on my list of friends, so I can't take credit of feeding this topic to them, but who knows who reads what post and when? Anyway, keep reading this for more scoops, I hope. temp today 98.6

Journal of the Plague Year, Day 134. Last week the DOH came into my ALF and tested 56 residents for COVID, about half the people who live there. The results are in and all 56 are negative. That's a big relief, especially when we don't know for sure how many asymptomatic cases there are in the population. We even had asymptomatic cases at our place. Now that we're cleared on this point we still have a lot to do. The DOH will come in and do a survey of policies and procedures that we are using to control COVID. As I've mentioned before, most of our policies meet or far exceed state standards so we think we will be ok unless they think up something new to impose. Once that's done visitors can come in, but lots of rules and regs on that too, that I'll describe in a future post as soon as I figure out what they are. temp today 98.0

Journal of the Plague Year, Day 135. today I was in a Zoom conference with the department of Geriatrics at Sinai, where I have a loose affiliation. These Zoom conferences are getting more and more efficient. The topic was blood clots caused by COVID19. Other corona viruses, as far as I know, don't produce this type of reaction, forming blood clots all over the body that can lead to strokes, heart attacks and a bunch of other unexpected problems. this is very different and very unexpected and very interesting. I hate interesting problems.

Give me a nice simple infection every time. Interesting problems are often followed by death. This virus appears different from others and so our discoveries and our treatments will be a lot different. There will be a lot more unexpected discoveries in the future. We're only about 6 months into this. I'll try and let you know about findings from the grass roots, but don't be surprised with what you'll be reading in the papers. I'll try and make sense of them as they roll out. temp today 98.4

Journal of the Plague Year, Day 136. On yesterday's Zoom meeting with the Geriatrics department at Sinai, I heard something new. Several docs reported that at the height of the COVID crises with ERs so crowded with virus cases that almost anyone going there was at high risk for catching it, even if they didn't have it, some EMS workers were refusing to take people to the ER even when the person asked to go. I've never heard that before. One of the docs said that it was illegal to refuse. What probably happened was that the ERs had such a reputation as dangerous places that the EMS people evaluated the patients in their homes, felt they were low risk, and took it on themselves to tiage the patients by not bringing them in. EMS staff are usually fearless in terms of their own risk but this is new. At that time, March and April, ER danger was so high that many patients, including some of mine, who really needed to be in the ER absolutely refused to go. Family members refused to send in loved ones. Docs, including me, really went out of our way to avoid sending people to ERs. Now that things are almost back to pre-COVID levels, people are going in much more easily, but this is just a picture of how the virus scarred even the most experienced front line health care providers. temp today 98.2

Journal of the Plague Year, Day 137. Another picture of the city's return seen from the underground. On Friday I was taking the subway home at about 5 o'clock. Recently the subway has been getting a little more crowded, even on the downtown trains I take. There were enough people in the car that everyone was about a foot or two from each other. Nobody was 6 feet apart, but nobody was touching shoulders either. The only absence was at 42nd street. Normally this stop is packed with office workers at 5, along with tourists and maybe a few people heading to the theater early. Now it was pretty empty. Few people getting on, few getting off. On the weekends when I take a taxi during my bar hopping trip around lower Manhattan the drivers always tell me that midtown is dead. These office workers, tourists and theater goers just aren't around, above ground taking taxis, or below ground in the subways. So as the downtown bar and restaurants open up and are getting more crowded, midtown business is still empty. It will take more time. How much? Who knows? temp today 97.7

Journal of the Plague Year, Day 140 (another numbering mistake yesterday. I forgot to number the weekend days so yesterday should have been 139 and today 140. OK, a little OCD behavior but as long as I'm doing this, might as well be accurate). Yesterday's post about the subways described what was changing with more people but empty Times Square station. One more thing seems the same. The overwhelming majority of people on the subways are minorities. Maybe it's because they have essential jobs and have to come in but can't work remotely from home like the office workers of midtown. I never really took a close notice of who rode the subways before, subways riders were subway riders. But when this is over I'm going to take a closer look and see if my initial unofficial subway census of a lot of interracial mixing on the subway was accurate or not, at least from 96th to 14th street. It's one of he things you don't pay attention to when something is as routine as daily commuting. temp today 97.7

Journal of the Plague Year, Day 141. 7-9 pounds! How could this be? In just 5 months since March I've been slowly gaining weight. A little is inactivity from quarantine. But most is from comfort food and stress eating from the whole quarantine, work, a change in jobs from Mount Sinai to a private group, change in benefits from Sinai to Medicare and private retirement funds. And when you stress eat and want comfort foods, sometimes tossed salads won't be enough. My accounts of bar/restaurant hopping around lower Manhattan on Sundays gives a little detail to this caloric journey. Well, it's time to go back to salads or something besides industrial strength Italian food. Maybe calamari from Rhode Island (the state with the highest per cent of Italian Americans in the country) or something like that. I'll let you know how it goes. temp today 98.2

Journal of the Plague Year, Day 142. FB is going into a new format before I even master the old one, other than simple posts. So, if things are harder to understand or follow, it wasn't my idea. After whining about weight gain yesterday, I have to confess one of my weaknesses. (Yes, although I'm an-ex catholic I still have a urge now and then to confess an occasional sin. Once a catholic always a catholic?) Since the start of COVID in March the ALF where I work has sometimes given us free lunches. At first it was paid for by the facility and often grateful family members of our residents. Money ran out after a while but this week it started up again with food supplied by NY State government and also paid for by the newly formed Food 1st Foundation, a non-profit set up by a major real estate company. Why all this? Employers, families, businesses, and government agencies want to show appreciation to first line health care workers and give them the morale support they need at times. These little perks of a free lunch now and then is great for morale, sometimes bad for the waistline (see yesterday's post), and appreciated by those on the receiving end. temp today. 98.0

Journal of the Plague Year, Day 143. We are starting to plan for the flu season. Most years community health nurses from Mount Sinai Hospital come to our facility in November and in one day give flu shots to almost all the patients and staff, including myself. I make sure they all see me getting my flu shot while they are getting theirs. This year we will try and do the same. We don't know how this is going to interact with COVID. In theory, both flu and COVID hitting the general population at the same time will increase the death rate. In fact, the death rate of them together could be higher than each one alone. In other words, if flu kills 30,000 and COVID is expected to kill 300,000 by the end of the year, the simultaneous epidemics might kill 400 or 500,000 instead of 330,000. On the other hand, isolation procedures for COVID might inhibit the spread of flu. We've haven't used isolation and distancing for flu, only vaccines, so maybe these new methods will keep the flu, and the flu-COVID combination, lower than expected. We'll see. temp today 98.2

Journal of the Plague Year, Day 146, Monday August 24. Recovery is uneven. As I walk around the neighborhood I see well established popular restaurants still closed and smaller less well known and sometimes just opened restaurants open and functioning. Why some and not others? I realized another anomaly last night. Fresh Direct, where you order on line and they deliver to your home was completely swamped in March. Every delivery slot was filled for weeks. Eventually it opened up and I'm able to order again. But they're out of stock of a lot of items including some of my favorites, and some of the low calorie healthy items. Out of 66 on my list of favorites, 25 have been unavailable for months. I don't know what's happening to their suppliers, or to them, but it seems like their recovery has been frozen in place for months. In comparison, my local D'Agostino's, Faicco's butcher shop, bagel shop, deli, and bodega are all back up to almost normal. Why some and not others? If opening up can be this variable, I think who survives will also be variable, and unpredictable. temp today. 98.2

Journal of the Plague Year, Day 147. More on the slow, slow reopening. NY is starting to allow visitors, like family members, into ALFs, but with a lot of requirements. Much of the policies and procedures at our place have been working since the start of this (isolation, quarantine for those exposed or sick, as much PPE as possible) but there is additional staff training the DOH wants. Also, new policies on visitors. They can only be a few at a time, have to meet under observed conditions, and have to give phone number and name so that if contact tracing is needed they can be found without too much trouble. This is the same thing that Astor Haircutters did months ago when I went for a haircut. Strange to give my phone number to my barber, but it was all for safety. There are probably a lot more rules I don't know about yet, but with a little luck we might be able to start taking visitors soon. We'll see. temp today 98.8

Journal of the Plague Year, Day 148. Most of my posts have been cautious if not downright pessimistic. Maybe a little optimism to change the tone. On day 103 of this series, Sunday July 12th, I wrote about tightly packed crowds of mask-less people were hanging out on Orchard street and I wondered if this was going to be the cause of another wave of infections. Although 45 days might not be a long enough period, there is still a little bit of hope that this isn't happening. There has been no significant increase in cases in NYC and we still have low enough numbers that the schools and restaurants can partially open. If this holds up, we'll be at a low enough level to handle the next two possible second waves. One will be when the kids are in school, maybe infecting each other and their teachers and parents, and probably when the flu season hits in December to March. But, so far so good, at least in New York. temp today. 98.3

Journal of the Plague Year, Day 149. One of the things I enjoy doing with these posts is to let people know about something that is occurring on a low level in day to day events that the mainline media or others haven't picked up on. I do the same thing with some of the articles I write for my neighborhood paper West View News (westviewnews.org) and I love it when we can scope the NY Times. On day 143 I wrote about the importance of getting flu shots this year to try and get some protection against a double whammy of flu and COVID. Today in my email I got an expected confirmation of what I wrote. Every week the head of the NY Dept of Health, Dr. Zucker, sends out a letter about some health related problem or issue that needs to be addressed. Today's letter was about the importance of vaccinations, including flu shots, in the upcoming few months. He also discussed vaccines for kids, which should also be done. The points about the possible flu/COVID wave that will probably come up this season is just about the same things I said a few days ago. If you had read my post then you can say that you saw it here first. Well, actually, this has been in the news for a while so neither I nor Zucker can completely take credit for some great discovery. But, it's still good to see your opinions confirmed by the head of the NY DOH. temp today. 98.3

Journal of the Plague Year, Day 150. Another possible sign of the city opening up: cars again. When this started in March all the streets were virtually empty at all times. I could cross West Street, aka the West Side Highway for us old timers, against the light and have nothing to worry about. Last weekend I couldn't cross West street due to traffic. Today when I was walking down Bleecker street at 5 PM I reached 7th avenue and it was packed with backed up traffic as far as the eye could see looking South. As with any traffic jam in the Village, there were cars trying to go through the side streets to go South, possibly to get to the Holland tunnel. None of this would be remarkable in normal times. But, this was the first time I've seen this during the COVID shut down. I also looked on the TV news and internet and couldn't see any report of an accident at the tunnel. So, one more tiny sign of things getting back to normal. Crowded, but normal. temp today 98.7

Journal of the Plague Year, Day 151, September 1. Hooray! The first day of Burning Man. I'm so glad I reserved the RV well in advance, and had an inside track to tickets, and got somebody to cover me at work, and found a good camp, Kostume Kult, to camp with. What could go wrong? Wait. What. A virus? How could this happen? Just a few years ago we figured out how to control Ebola, so how could this slip through?

OK, enough fantasy. Today would have been the first day of Burning Man. (If you don't know about it go to burningman.org or multiple Youtube videos for a relatively cleaned up description of the festival.) But it doesn't take much to see that the problems of 75.000 people doesn't amount to a hill of beans in this crazy world. (Yes, that line is stolen from the end scene of Casablanca). But, it's true. Almost every day, including today, I learn of someone else who was sick or who died from COVID. The warmth and open air of Burning Man might have made things a little safer, but when 75,000 or so people are sitting shoulder to shoulder for several hours that's just asking for trouble. Masks, distance, quarantine, it's all so simple and so low tech, and all so necessary. And, we're not done with this yet. temp. today 98.8

Journal of the Plague Year, Day 152. Most of these posts have to do with my own experiences during the COVID age rather than take something from the news and analyze it. But today there was a story that links me, Burning Man (see yesterday's post) and COVID. There is a community of Burners, as we call ourselves, in NYC. One of the places we gather is a bar called Lucky on Ave B in the East Village. The owner is Abby a long time Burner. I read in the papers today that she is suing the state over the rules on bars. The rules say that bars must also serve food with alcohol and not just drinks. Lucky has never had food, and for them to bring in food just to turn it around and sell it with alcohol is foolish. But, those are the state rules, unless Abby wins her suit. I'm not sure if C****, or whoever made the rule, thought that food and drink would somehow be better than drink alone and somehow make our control of COVID related behavior more sedate. A dive bar is a dive bar, and I say that in the best sense of the word, especially one with a nice back yard like Lucky should be allowed to operate as it did before. There are enough restaurants and bars around the city that won't survive this lock down already. I'm also hoping that some scientist somewhere in the world can prove that Guiness protects against COVID. One can always hope. temp today. 98.3

Journal of the Plague Year, Day 153. One more post about Burning Man with an additional moral to the story. When Burning Man announced it would not meet in person, but only virtually, Burners started working on various videos. The are scattered over the internet and Youtube, some with animations some with people, some mixes. They give a good idea of what the event would have been, without being in 100 degree heat and dust storms. You can also see that it's a lot of artistic types, both creative arts and performing arts, and lots of New Age people. Not just filled with ex-sixties hippies. And, no contact means no COVID spread. Compare this to the Sturgis motorcycle rally where several hundred thousand people gathered in person, no masks because they're just so butch. Now there have been cases of COVID traced to the event and the surrounding states have had sharp increases in cases. I'm not sure how many have died so far, but many will die as infections from this super spreader event spread throughout the entire country. I miss Burning Man, but I'm sure loved ones of the Sturgis bikers who died from COVID will miss them a lot more. temp today 97.9

Journal of the Plague Year, Day 154. When these posts started I complained about a cancelled convention, the American Medical Directors Society, which is a meeting of nursing home and assisted living medical directors. It would have been during the first week of April in Chicago and attracts thousands. Even though it was early in the pandemic, it was obvious it couldn't be held in person and so the whole thing was done by Zoom or WebEx and put on videos. I just got a chance to go through the videos and actually it was pretty good as a learning experience. I was able to stop the videos and repeat parts, look up unfamiliar terms, or just see the videos when I was wide awake. Conventions are great for learning, but also for seeing friends and hitting the bars and restaurants in a mini-vacation in another city. With videos, none of this. But, I still miss in person conventions and hope they come back soon. temp today. 98.3

Journal of the Plague Year, Day 155 (a little late). Friday was a good day for a modest step toward normality. The state allowed visitors to assisted living facilities (I'm not sure about nursing homes) so they could see their loved ones. Two families came to visit under the following rules.

They had to make an appointment a day ahead of the visit, only two visitors at a time, they had to wear masks and sit 6 feet apart from the person they visited. No hugging. Visits were 45 minutes and during the visit there had to be a staff member observing the visit so they wouldn't break the rules. The visitors who came today sat in our large back yard, obeying the rules, with a staff member at the other side of the yard where he could observe the visit, but be too far away to hear what was said and so allow privacy of conversation. There will be more visits soon and I hope they go as smoothly as these two did. Maybe even hugging some day. temp today 98.7

Journal of the Plague Year, Day 159, Tuesday September 8. A few days ago I described the medical convention I attended on line. It was presented in early April so some of the stuff was a few months old. One topic that came out again was the use of telemedicine. A doctor can stay at home and have the patient at the other end of a Zoom interview. Maybe the patient is alone, maybe with a staff member with them, if they are both in the medical office, even when the doc isn't. When COVID started, I didn't even consider. First, I figured this was part of my job no matter what. Doctors have gone to work in epidemics much worse than COVID. Besides, there's no comparison between seeing a person live vs over a computer line, at least in my opinion. Also, the technical aspects are a pain, learning new billing rules, new regulations, and a dozen other details. At the start of the epidemic lots of doctors did this. Over time, this has opened up with some doctors back to in person visits and some still on line, and some with a mixture of both. I have enough problems maneuvering around this FaceBook page let alone learning an entire new tech. Also, if I stayed home and worked over the internet, what would the other staff who have to come in, like the personal aides, nurses, therapists, etc,, especially those with kids, do. COVID has disrupted things enough. If the rest of the staff didn't see me coming in, how could they keep doing it. temp today 98.2

Journal of the Plague Year, Day 160. A friend asked me about voting in nursing homes and assisted living facilities. I don't know about nursing homes, or even other ALFs but I can describe what's happening at my place. In previous elections, the Board of Elections would send a staff member to meet with residents of the ALF, register those unregistered, and showing people how to fill out the absentee ballots. All residents at the ALF have some pre-existing condition or another and so all can qualify for absentee ballots even before COVID. It was done in the activity room as a group event. Now we are on partial quarantine. The BOE doesn't have staff to send us. So, our recreation therapist is taking applications for ballots to each registered voter individually and when the ballots come back she will show them how to fill it out and send it back. It's roughly the same amount of voting, but taking a lot more effort to do it. Medical visits, rehab visits, exercise classes, medication delivery, meal delivery, etc are all in the same boat. Every service is being delivered but it takes much more time to do it. That's with a somewhat reduced staff. I just hope we can keep this up in the months to come. temp today. 98.6

Journal of the Plague Year, Day 161. Last week I crossed state lines for a relief from COVID. I got together with friends from graduate school at the Blue Eyes Cafe on Sinatra blvd in Sinatra park. Frank Sinatra (look him up Millennials) grew up in Hoboken so the town is loaded with little memorials to him. It sits on the banks of the Hudson River and has a beautiful view of Manhattan. We get together periodically in Jersey or Manhattan, or sometimes Bronxville. After a nice Italian meal they surprised me by treating me to the meal as a way of thanking me for doing my job. I felt a little guilty accepting it, but not guilty enough to refuse. Take your perks where you can get them. Thanks again friends. temp today 98.7

Journal of the Plague Year, Day 162. A small scene on the street. I passed a bus parked on Fifth Avenue yesterday. The door was open and the driver was shouting out, "Work with me here, put your mask on." I didn't stop to gawk at the confrontation but afterward I started to wonder where this confrontation was heading. If the person put on the mask, it was over and settled. If not, the driver could refuse to move the bus until he/she did, delaying everyone else and putting him behind schedule for his route. Or, he could have called a cop. This being on Fifth Avenue and 109th street they would probably respond relatively quickly. I don't know exactly what authority cops have; giving a ticket, removing from the bus, arresting, or what. But, if the person continued to refuse then the cops would be face with the job of removing the person or just ignoring the infraction, which defeats the purpose of having rules about masks. Home tonight I saw an article about a bus driver attacked by two people he kicked off his bus for some infraction (thevillagesun.com). They were later arrested. I don't know how many times across the country these low level confrontations occur, but Youtube and the evening news seems to have plenty of them. For now, I wear my mask every time and every place out of my apartment. And, I don't ride buses, subways are now filled with masked people. temp today 98.0

Journal of the Plague Year, Day 165, Monday September 14. Yesterday after dinner I took a taxi home and, as usual, I asked the driver how business was. He appeared to be Chinese with a thick accent and I couldn't understand everything, but he started talking about mid-town being dead and the only business was in lower Manhattan, and the upper East and West sides. He said that's where the restaurants are open and that's where the people are. He then hoped that they didn't open like Florida did. He said because the governor listened to T**** and the bars and restaurants were wide open, that's where the deaths are occurring now. (one of yesterday's waitresses supported this, and I'll discuss in a future post). He knew that 25% indoor seating wasn't enough to help. More on that in a future post also. Like the old 1930s movies when some wise talking cab driver, usually with a Brooklyn accent, seems to know a lot about what is going on, this guy went on for the whole ride about what it would take to turn things around. In spite of some people denying the seriousness of the situation, enough people do know what's going on. Let's hope that helps somehow. temp today 98.4

Journal of the Plague Year, Day 166. These posts vary from very hopeful to very pessimistic. Today's is mixed. I wrote earlier about the possibility of the COVID and flu hitting us at the same time and making everything so much worse that either one alone. An article in Science magazine, August 28, looked at flu season in the Southern Hemisphere where it hits before it hits us. In Argentina, Chile, Australia, and South Africa this year's flu cases were only about one per cent of what it was last year, although last year was a somewhat bad year. The theory is that precautions against COVID and cut down on flu transmission since they are both respiratory viruses spread roughly the same way. I don't know how careful COVID precautions were down there (masks, social distance, quarantine) but this is a little hopeful that maybe the parts of the US that have instituted adequate precautions might lessen the double whammy of COVID/flu. Let's hope. temp today 97.7

Journal of the Plague Year, Day 167. On day 155 I described the rules for visitors coming to the ALF to see loved ones. They have to reserve ahead of time, can only stay 45 minutes, wear masks, stay 6 feet apart and have to have a staff member nearby observing that they obey the rules. These rules seem to take a lot of the fun and spontaneous nature of the visit away. So after the first few visits, how have the visitors responded? They stopped coming. The opted for the alternative which is to come and take their loved one out on a day trip or overnight stay over. The state rules allow for 1-2 day leave of absence from the facility for the resident without any problems. So now they come, take their family member or friend out of the building for a few hours to a few days and they can stay out long, stay close, hug or kiss, avoid face masks, and not have to be chaperoned by a staff member. It's much more enjoyable. Let's hope it's not too enjoyable and one of the visitors doesn't have an asymptomatic case of COVID. Rules and rigidity might be safer and flexibility is more enjoyable. That's the trade off. Let's hope it doesn't cause problems. temp. today 96.8

Journal of the Plague Year, Day 168. I've tried to balance good news and bad news. Sometimes they overlap and sometimes the good news is very fragile with a thin margin of safety. My ALF had 100% negative COVID tests among staff and 50% of residents who agreed to be tested. All good, we were allowed to have visitors (see yesterdays post as to how this played out), and no COVID infected people. But, recently this was put at risk. Our nurses aren't allowed to do skilled nursing, like complicated wound care. We have to call in a CHHA nurse (Certified Home Healthcare Agency) to do it. Recently, one of these nurses tested positive and so it looked like the state was going to put the entire facility on the quarantine list with a lock down order. Fortunately, the state agreed that since this nurse wasn't around the facility all the time, and only to come and treat one patient, it was sufficient for the CHHA nurse and the one patient she was seeing to both be on isolation for 14 days to see if they became sick. 14 days have passed and both patient and nurse are ok. So, we've dodged the bullet. But, it was close and the state department of health, the DOH, could have taken a hard line that we would have had to obey. They were flexible and we all benefited. But, it was close. temp today. 97.3

Journal of the Plague Year, Day 169. You hear people say that disasters sometimes brings out the best in people. It also sometimes brings out the worst. One of my minor pleasures is to sleep late on days I'm not working, maybe to noon. With quarantine, the newspapers that were delivered to my door every morning, the NY Daily News and NY Times had to be left down in a little alcove of the lobby instead of my door. I noticed that now and then The Times would be missing, especially if I got up late or waited until I got home from work to take it upstairs. The doorman said that others had complained of the same. One of my neighbors in our co-op was using this situation to sometimes steal our papers. Now, on the days I really want them, like the weekends, I have to get up early at 8 or so and get down to the lobby to retrieve my papers. If I wait until 10:30, it could be gone. My building is expensive so anyone who can afford to live here should be able to afford a subscription to The Times if it is so important. Considering everything that's going on, if losing a newspaper now and then is the worst that happens to me during this lockdown, or having to get up early on a weekend morning, I'll be very happy. Trivial problems like this are trivial, or as Saturday Night Live used to describe "White People's Problems." Besides leaving a note next to the stack of papers, which didn't stop the situation, next I'll try to get them to return the paper after they read it. That way stealing is changed to borrowing. Much more agreeable. temp today 98.2

Journal of the Plague Year, Day 172, Monday September 21. Yesterday I was on Mulberry Street in Little Italy at Cafe Palermo having an espresso, sambuca, and pastry. I was speaking to somcone who worked on the San Gennaro fcstival. It was supposed to start two Thursdays ago, but COVID cancelled big events like that. They did have a procession of the saint's statue but no large crowds or food/game stalls like before. I go every year and I missed it. He pointed out that this would have been a fantastically successful feast since it didn't rain one day during the 11 day span. Rain is one of the things that hurts the finances of the feast a lot and 11 clear days would have been great. A missed feast, like a few missed newspapers, isn't the worst thing that can happen in the midst of an epidemic, but it just seems that having 11 perfect days for a missed feast is just making things so much more frustrating. It's almost like fate was teasing us. Maybe it was. temp today 97.2

Journal of the Plague Year, Day 173. I've tried to make every post about COVID. Today's different. Today at my ALF a smoke alarm went off and it turned out to be real, not one of the usual false alarms or fire drills. Several cable systems come into our building and one overheated down in the basement where my office is. A dozen of us had to sequester at the other end of the hall until the fire department determined that there was no real fire, just smoke and overheating. The nurses and aides didn't even have enough time to flirt with the firemen. Eventually, the two cable companies we use for all cable TV and computer lines, and Con Edison sent in people to check the lines to prevent this happening again. There is no direct COVID relationship to this brief event, except that when bad things are happening there can always be more bad things coming down the road. Like yesterday's San Gennaro feast being cancelled during one of the most perfect 11 days of weather we've had in a long time, this is another case of fate pilling on bad news. But, no flaming inferno so I guess a smoky cable closet is a lot better than it could have been. temp today 98.0

Journal of the Plague Year, Day 174. One of the major parts of NYC that is struggling to return to normal is the restaurant business. They often operate on a narrow margin with lots of failures even before COVID, and now is worse. One recent rule change is to allow indoor dining at 25% capacity starting around October 1st. The two restaurant owners I know had the following opinions: "It won't do shit for us." and "it will kill us". Why? For one thing 25% would not make a big difference in income. But, with indoor dining comes lots of rules such as distancing, ventilation, cleaning between customers, etc. Breaking any of these rules could result in citations for minimal income benefits. But, if some restaurants are doing it, there will be a pressure for all restaurants and bars to do it and those who can't do it easily will still be forced to try. It's hard to predict how strictly rules will be enforced while getting a few extra tables but getting cited and possibly losing your liquor license because of those citations is a high price. temp today 97.9

Journal of the Plague Year, Day 175 (a little late). Another thing the city is doing to help restaurants is to allow them a 10% COVID surcharge on their bills without being accused to price gouging. But the two restaurant owners I spoke to are both passing on this surcharge. They think that it will cut down on tips for the staff. they aren't sure if it will cut down business considering how expensive food in Manhattan is anyway, but they are pretty sure tips will suffer. One waitress I spoke to wasn't so sure either way. In any case, this is one more way the city is trying to help restaurants but just can't figure out an easy way to do it. temp today 98.1

Journal of the Plague Year, Day 176. Possible good news for NYC restaurants. Outdoor eating will be permanent, at least for now. How this will work in practice isn't clear. As usual, there will also be a lot of regulations. Heating with propane gas or electric heaters will be allowed, although where they can be used (sidewalk or street traffic lane) will be regulated. More seats will be opened but the total still has to obey the 25% capacity rule, at least for now. Hope is that it will slowly increase to higher percents. When I lived in LA they did this a lot with clear plastic barriers around the outdoor seats and heaters of one type or another for comfort. It worked well but LA winters weren't like NYC winters. Also, these toys are expensive and LA had years to do something that NYC restaurants and bars have to do in a month or two. We'll see. temp today 97.5

Journal of the Plague Year, Day 179, Monday September 28. I last posted about what might happen to restaurants with the new permanent outdoor seats. After asking around to the places I go, I can see what is starting to happen. One place has outdoor seats spread around on an open sidewalk and putting up plastic curtains and heaters would be tough. Two others with wooden barriers surrounding their tables and tables that are tightly packed could put an enclosure around them and space heaters for warmth. Meanwhile, restaurant owners are demonstrating in front of Cuomo's office asking him to increase indoor dining from 25% capacity to 50. But people will have to decide soon. As they said in the TV show, "Winter is coming." temp today 98.4

Journal of the Plague Year, Day 180. Progress against COVID is coming, but very slowly. A few weeks ago the state sent us COVID testing materials that can give an answer in 15 minutes. But, we had to get the approval of a lab that could supervise the tests, or something like that. We had to sign a form taking responsibility for the tests accuracy and somehow coordinate with the lab even though the test material was self contained and didn't need to go to the lab to be processed. So we signed and waited for the lab to acknowledge the affiliation. Today I learned we signed the wrong form, so we got a different one (hopefully the right one this time) and signed it. It seems like every step we take is clumsy and slow. I hope we get all these details worked out soon. Unfortunately some areas of NYC are having COVID spikes so we may end up having more time to fight this out than what we thought. temp today 99.0

Journal of the Plague Year, Day 181. Today was the first day of indoor dining in NYC, even though only 25%. Piccolo Angolo, my favorite, had 5 tables instead of over 20. They had an indoor HEPA filter to clean the air, took my temp, name, address and contact info as required by regulations. They were also looking at how to protect some of their outdoor tables and were pricing electric heaters. I'll check out a few more places over the weekend. There was something else. What was that? Oh, yes, the spinach salad, house red, a Sangiovese, and fettucine alfredo were great (don't worry, I'm on Crestor). temp today 98.1

Journal of the Plague Year, Day 182. Going back and forth between job related COVID stuff to city related stuff (mostly restaurants and bars) is dizzying. Wish I could rearrange them in sequence. In any case, today we're back to work issues. A few days ago I mentioned my work place will be able to do on site fast (15 minutes) tests. More details. along with permission from the DOH came more regulations. All tests using this fast method have to be reported to a website that sends it to the state. We don't have our access to this site yet. Tests are only supposed to be on people who have symptoms, have been close to COVID positive people, and a half dozen other qualifications. This is going really slowly, and I'm not sure how many times we're going to do this even when approved, but every little step helps. temp today 98.4

Journal of the Plague Year, Day 183. Today is my birthday, 73 years old. It's as good a time as any to take a different tact in these posts. I've spoken about the virus from the viewpoint of what I've seen myself, at my job and around the city. Next week is the time for a different view. What is going on at the national policy level? Next week will be five full days of anti-T**** attacks. Even before he came down with the virus, in a cosmic level case of poetic justice, I was itching to do this. If you like T**** you might want to avoid these posts until October 13th (I'm taking off Columbus day), or get ready for some really nasty facts about his performance during this epidemic. Political arguments over the internet usually end with long back and forth chains of responses so I'll do as much as I can stomach. To get a taste of what I'll write you can go to westviewnews.org and look for my articles, especially "Is T**** guilty of homicide." temp today 97.2

Journal of the Plague Year, Day 186, Monday October 5. The first of five anti-T**** polemics. Let's start at the beginning. He started to get warnings about COVID in January, realized how dangerous it was by February with more data coming in from other countries all the time. And yet he couldn't help but lie to the people and say it was no worse than the flu, would disappear like a miracle, etc. He hoped he could fake it until November. He couldn't, the virus moved faster than his lies. But the worst part is that he said "nothing could be done" even now looking back at it. By March it was clear that testing, masks, social distancing, shut downs, and quarantine could dramatically cut down cases and deaths. If he had made a strong statement then in favor of these tools the spineless R********* governors would have all gone along and his deplorable (C****** words) and disgusting people (T**** own words) who worship him would have gone along also. He could have made obeying these rules a mark of patriotism and support for him and all his people would have followed and saved tens of thousands of lives. He even could have sold M*** face masks and made a fortune, and he was too stupid to even do that. temp today 98.4

Journal of the Plague Year, Day 187. T**** has done so many bad things in relation to COVID that we have to break it down into categories. The first is criminal negligence. This occurs when a person ignores obvious risks and behaves in a manner that most reasonable people would not. For example, if a parent ignores medical advice for standard medical care, and a loved one dies as a result, that might qualify. In other words, they didn't do what they should have done by common sense standards. When every epidemic specialist says actions should be taken like isolation, testing, masks, and quarantine and T**** ignores them, that's negligence. If people died, as they did, that might qualify as criminal negligence, a felony. I'm sure there have been cases where parents ignored medical advice, like using exorcism instead of medicine for a simple medical problem, and the child suffered or dies, they were held liable. Maybe they even lost custody of their other kids. T**** did this 200,000 times over. temp today 98.5

Journal of the Plague Year, Day 188. Criminal negligence is not doing what you should, and today's definition is of reckless endangerment where you do something that you shouldn't. You do something that is reckless and that most people under similar circumstances wouldn't. Having an indoor rally where people are discouraged from wearing masks or social distancing is an example. So is having an outdoor garden meeting where people are without masks and too close together even though you know a person nearby (Hicks) tested positive and you might be positive too. Coming back to the White House and exposing your staff to a deadly disease by not wearing a mask every minute of the day is reckless. People will get sick and some may die, like Herman Cain did. If a parent left a kid in the back seat of a car in the sun that parent would often be arrested immediately and the kid taken away to safety. But, when he puts thousands of his own supporters at risk he just gets cheers and applause. At least, until November 3. temp today 97.8

Journal of the Plague Year, Day 189. As bad as his previously described actions were, once T**** is out of office people can start working on doing things the right way and maybe minimizing or reversing the damage he has done. But there is one area where his damage might last long after he's gone. He has undermined the medical researchers at the CDC and FDA so that there opinions are now not respected. The CDC never had a scandal like this, and the FDA has been undermined by conservatives and lobbyists, but never to this extent. Once researchers lose their reputation or quit, it can't be recovered immediately. It takes a long time. In a country where there is already an anti-v** movement that can kill people the trust in future vaccines has dropped to an all time low among the public. Even when a COVID vaccine is available, many people will avoid it because they don't trust T**** and so they don't trust the people who worked under his "leadership" and won't trust their opinions. It will take years to re-establish trust. And that's just COVID. He's done the same undermining of global warming and environmental science which will eventually lead to catastrophic damage to the country. temp today 99.1 (it's not high, I just had pizza).

Journal of the Plague Year, Day 190. When this pandemic started we gave T**** the benefit of the doubt and just assumed he was too stupid to realize what was happening. Woodward's interviews showed this was wrong and he knew the dangers involved. He didn't care. He thought he could minimize the dangers, blame somebody else (O****, Chinese, WHO) or just bluff his way until Nov 3. Many people made mistakes at the beginning of the epidemic but others learned from their mistakes, changed behavior, and figured out the correct thing to do. He didn't want to look weak or admit a mistake so he doubled down and killed tens of thousands of people while doing so. Maybe hundreds of thousands before this is over.

And his enablers and followers will continue this after he is voted out. Sad. temp today 98.9

Journal of the Plague Year, Day 194, Tuesday October 13th. I watched the Hassidim in Brooklyn burning masks in the street to protest restrictions and it reminded me of the Nazi book burnings in the 1930s. All it needed was a few medical textbooks thrown into the fire to make the comparison complete. They were proud of obeying their own laws instead of the laws of the US. But, I don't think they were even obeying Jewish law. I went to medical school at Einstein which was run by the Orthodox Yeshiva University at that time. When medical decisions and religious teaching came into conflict (working on Shabbos, Kosher food, autopsies, DNR orders, etc) the ultimate rule was to preserve life. The preservation of life, according to Jewish law, was the ultimate obligation of a moral person. Of course, COVID deniers, Hassidic or otherwise, can get around this by just saying the science is wrong and masks, isolation, quarantine, smaller meetings, etc are not needed. When caring for patients at Einstein, Jewish or gentile, Orthodox or Reform you never heard this anti-science thinking. All you heard was "help me" or "help my loved one". But the guys (and they were all guys) burning masks and endangering health down in Midwood knew better than anyone. A shonda. temp today 98.5

Journal of the Plague Year, Day 195. Winter is here. This week, for the first time, I've seen outdoor heaters in front of some of the restaurants on Hudson street. My favorite place, Piccolo Angolo has an electric heater but hasn't been able to test it yet since the weather has been so good. Other places have propane heaters. But propane heaters require fire department permits. The have to certify that the heater is safe and not a fire hazard. It's unclear if the FDNY will give the restaurants a pass on these permits, require them but make them easy to obtain, or require them and enforce really strict regulations. Violations might result in citations again, like the ones that were used to pull liquor licenses from some bars and restaurants.

And, although they look like they might work if you have enough of them and the temp is 50 or 40, what happens when it goes down into the 30s with wind and snow? We'll see. temp today 98.9

Journal of the Plague Year, Day 196. Over the last week I had dinner twice at restaurants that had views of the sidewalk pedestrian traffic. Besides eating and drinking, I started to count the number of people walking by with and without masks. On Hudson street 30 without masks and 60 with. On Orchard street there were 27 without masks and 52 with. So about 1/3 of people in the downtown area were without masks. I don't know how this is going to translate into infections. According to the videos I have seen on the news, in areas of NYC where the virus is spreading, like some Brooklyn neighborhoods, very few people were wearing masks. Let's hope that's what it takes to spread the virus, because if you need that level of carelessness the spread it, then 1/3 maskless might be sufficient to contain it, as the low infection rate of Manhattan shows. Of course, 100% with masks would be so much safer. temp today. 97.9

Journal of the Plague Year, Day 197. When my cousins Bob and Maria came down to Hudson street a few weeks ago to share brunch, she noticed something I hadn't. The masses of young people filling the seats of the restaurants along Hudson were gorgeous! She said it was like a waiting room for a modeling agency. Walking around the neighborhood I realized she was right, "lookist" but right. But she said something else. "How can these young folks afford apartments in this neighborhood?" That took a little more thought. Either they have always been around, but indoors and invisible, or they are drawn into the area by the attractive trendy bars and restaurants. Maybe grey haired old farts like me just hang out in different places. This reminded my of when I lived in Los Angeles. That is the land of beautiful people, they say. When I was there and travelled around the city, the people looked like anywhere else; all sizes, shapes, races, attractiveness, ages, etc. But, on Venice Beach, and probably some of the beach towns south of L.A., the local denizens did look like Greek Gods and Goddesses (and not just Dionysus). What does this have to do with COVID? Well, maybe this pandemic has brought out stuff about our area that was right under our noses but some of us didn't notice. In upcoming posts I'll talk about other characteristics of our neighbors and friends that the plague has brought out, both good and bad. temp today 98.8

Journal of the Plague Year, Day 200, Monday October 19. As much as we would all like to have things get back to normal, sometimes measures to do this produce controversy. The city just allowed restaurants that have sidewalk and curbside tables to continue them permanently. This would help them plan and invest for long term improvement. But Community Board 2 which covers Greenwich Village had a recent meeting where there was a lot of opposition to this. Restaurants vs local residents has been a long term conflict in this area, mostly having to do with noise complaints and bars/restaurants staying open too late, even before work days. CB2 complaints focused on the excesses of restaurants occurring right now, like them controlling sidewalks like they were private property and over crowding in areas with multiple bars/restaurants. There will be a lot of fighting over this in the future. Strict enforcement can keep places in line or lose their liquor license, which is what happened to the White House Bar and resulted in them and other places along Hudson street controlling their crowds a lot better. Eventually, there might be push back to this anti-night life pushback if some well like neighborhood establishments going under. CB2 and others will be blamed for killing cherished establishments. Preserving our nightlife without further destroying our quality of life while helping desired establishments could become very complicated and heated. temp today 98.4

Journal of the Plague Year, Day 201. On Saturday I took the subway to go to dinner at about 5:30. It was packed. It's not uncommon for weekend subway rides to be crowded since they run so many less trains.

This was about as crowded as it used to get before COVID. Subway riders have been slowly increasing over the last few months. But this ride marked a milestone. It was the first time since March that the train was so crowded that my shoulder and leg touched the person sitting next to me. That's not a big deal in itself, but it does show a tiny move to normalcy. And this was on a Saturday, the day for shoppers, tourists, and diners. During the week numbers have gone up too, but more on this tomorrow. temp today 99.0

Journal of the Plague Year, Day 202. Still trying to get the pulse of the city from the underground. I mentioned yesterday that the Saturday subway crowd looked pretty "normal". Today and yesterday I paid more attention to the workweek subway crowd. More people than in March-April but not normal yet. A lot of people got onto the subway at 42nd street in the AM rush and they almost all got out at 96th, the last stop to transfer to the 1 train Broadway local. On the way back at 5 PM the train was full, not packed and a lot of people got off at 42nd street. But almost nobody got on at 42nd. I think this is due to empty office buildings and missing tourists. These quarantiners have not returned, at least going by this indirect measurement. I don't know how many people this represents throughout the city. Also, as far as I can judge, the riders are still over represented by minorities, even during the 96th to 42nd street stretch. At the start of all this I thought whites were missing, and I still think so. When it is really all over and everything comes back to normal I'll pay more attention to the ethnicity of my fellow subway riders so by then maybe I'll know if this is all in my imagination or is a real slice of the city. We'll see. temp today 98.1

Journal of the Plague Year, Day 203. A few days ago I saw the first graffiti on the side of one of the sidewalk enclosures on Christopher street. It said "Pito" which I assume is somebody's nick name. The only translation I could find in Romance languages is "whistle" in Spanish. There are enclosures all over the city now so that's a lot of virgin canvases for artists to decorate. Owners of these enclosures might be tempted to allow artists a free hand at decoration. Be careful. Artists who produce outstanding work might claim propriety ownership over the restaurant owner. There is a case in the courts I believe where an artist claimed works done on plywood boards that the owner of the boards, a restauranteur, claims for himself. The 5 Pointz development in Queens was covered in outstanding art work and when it was demolished the developer was forced to pay 6.7 million to the artists for violating public art. So, owners, be careful about what prior agreements you have, if any, and how long you let street art exist before covering it. And, when disassembling your enclosures, dispose of them properly, if you can figure out exactly how. temp today 98.2

Journal of the Plague Year, Day 204. Living in my own co-op apartment has made me miss one of the major consequences of the plague. Speaking to a waiter and a waitress last week during diner woke me up. Initial rents are starting to drop dramatically in some areas. One waitress said that around Union Square where she lives rents have only dropped a few hundred dollars, but the apartments that are available are much much larger than hers. A waiter from Bed-Stuy in Brooklyn said that the previous range of rents were $1500-1700 but now are going down to about $1000 with some studios as low as $700. I don't know if I got this from one of them or from the papers but in midtown areas where rents are $4000, they have dropped to $2500. If this is happening in Manhattan and Bed-Stuy it might be happening in a lot more neighborhoods, especially hot ones with overpriced ridiculous rents. This will reverse once the plague is over, but for now it looks like this is real and wide spread. I don't know if businesses are having the same changes, but I'll try and find out. temp today 98.2

Addendum to last night's post. New York One on Spectrum had a piece a few hours after my post about the same thing. they interviewed several residents about having hard times and getting rent reductions. And they also mentioned that landlords, especially small ones, are also having a hard time making ends meet. everyone is scrambling to figure out how to survive. more on this next week.

Journal of the Plague Year, Day 207, Monday October 26. There has been a lot of talk about people leaving NYC in droves. Is it true? I live in a co-op in the far West Village with a little over 70 apartments. I asked my doorman how many people were out of town and not in their apartments and he said about 10. But, he added that's about what it usually is this time of year. It's not really that different. Other Facers who are in this group living in NYC, ask around. Is this flight from NYC a myth or what? Also, they newspaper articles almost always talk about people fleeing to The Hamptons. They seem to think every New Yorker has a second home out there. They never mention the Jersey Shore or Cape Cod, but I know New Yorkers do go there, and to upstate NY or other states also. It's not just billionaires going to Florida. And, when the virus is contained, whenever that will be, the majority will come back to NYC like we did after 9/11 or hurricane Sandy. temp today 98.7

Journal of the Plague Year, Day 208. Last week the residents and staff at the ALF where I work got flu shots. Some things were the same as before with almost all the staff and the overwhelming majority of residents getting their flu shot, including me. But instead of doing it in one room where everyone saw every else getting shots, in sort of a communal event, our CEO who is a nurse went up to each apartment and gave everyone their shots individually. It took twice as long, but it got done. Nobody knows if this year's flu season will be horrible because COVID is hitting us at the same time, or if it will be better because protections against COVID (masks, quarantine, etc) will also protect against the flu. We might not know this for another few months, but the path has been set for us. temp today 98.2

Journal of the Plague Year, Day 209. Another small piece of progress has come from the state. Previously, all group activities were banned, but now they are allowing small group meetings of, I believe, ten or fewer people, appropriately spaced. We have decided to use our library where there is sufficient space to have activities. They will include current even discussion groups, exercise classes, yoga, maybe tai chi, pet therapy (even demented patients know how to pet a dog) and others. Before COVID we could have 2-3 activities a day with 20-30 people in each activity. Now we will have 2 a day with 10 people max each. The question is, so far, will people come to these activities because they are climbing the walls and want to get more active, or will they avoid the meetings because they are scared of COVID, no matter what the state says. This same question might come up again as restaurants open up and are allowed to do 50% or more of capacity. Will people show up? We'll see. temp today 98.0

Journal of the Plague Year, Day 210. Every few days I learn of another place closing but the opposite is also happening. I've written a lot about the bars/restaurants of Hudson, Bleecker, Orchard and Mulberry streets. I realized that with all the closings and potential closings, there are a hard core of places that are absolutely determined to stay open. When take home was allowed, they started immediately. Sidewalk tables, when allowed, went up within a week as did tables in the curbside traffic lane when it opened. The city then said you needed platforms in the street for the tables and they went up immediately. Then, an 18 inch separation from active traffic lanes and a combination of woodwork and planters popped up. When year long outdoor dining was announced the tables were turned into well built sheds and heaters went up. 25% occupancy? No problem, even though "...this won't do shit for us." They opened anyway. Every step of opening was immediately grasped by these hard core survivors. I hope they make it, even though there are still casualties every week. temp today 98.6

Journal of the Plague Year, Day 211. Yesterday I talked about restaurants fight to survive. today we look at Delis. In my immediate neighborhood there are many, but I'll look at five in particular. On one block on

Hudson there is a Starbucks, open til about 6, usually lines in front early in morning, thin out during the day. At the other end is Black Stone Coffee Roasters which is a gourmet type deli, with tables outside and a line in the early hours. In the middle is Hudson Gourmet Deli, which is where I go. Open 24/7, run by an Egyptian family that is desperately working to keep it solvent. 24/7 is a tough schedule but they do it. Never have a long line like the other places but they keep working. On Christopher there is Hudson Bagels, also run by mostly Egyptians. I go there also. Around the corner from me is a bodega run by a Dominican family, reduced hours but still going. I go there also. If you want a place to stay open you have to patronize it. I'm only one person and I can only eat a certain number of bagels and bacon/egg/cheese sandwiches. But I try my best. I don't know how many of these will survive, but I know all five are working hard. And, there are a half dozen other places within walking distance, working just as hard. good luck to all of them. temp today 97.6

Journal of the Plague Year, Day 214, Monday November 2. A few weeks ago I had a nice brunch in a local restaurant, Philip Marie. This week I found out it was closing for good. Another COVID victim? Two restaurant owners I know, and who knew Philip Marie said it was more complicated. One said he had trouble with the landlord before and he wasn't willing to cut a deal. Another said he had the place for a long time and was ready to retire. It reminded me that COVID is not the only problem small business owners have been having recently. Before COVID there was plenty of concern about small businesses of all types, especially related to rising rents, and many closed. COVID has made things worse, but not unique. Small places always have a hard time and opening a small business of any type is always a big risk in terms of time, money and emotional investment. One good note. On the blackboard of Philip Marie was the touching message "Thanks for the memories, Until we meet again. Food, Wine, Love", the last three words being their motto over the years. temp today 97.8

Journal of the Plague Year, Day 215. For the first time in about nine months I had dinner indoors with 3 friends. We were at the National Arts Club where they are members. It looks like an old fashion type "gentleman's club" from the 1800s but takes in men and women as members and they should all have some connection with art. The dinner was great, as was the wine, and it was good to be indoors again, with appropriate social distancing and masking. After that, went home for a nice relaxing evening watching TV, but there were a lot of specials on about, I assume, the geography of the US since all they had up were maps of the country. I like geography as much as anyone but couldn't they find something more exciting to talk about? Maybe something more interesting will happen tomorrow. So, after a nice relaxed quiet evening temp today is 98.1

Journal of the Plague Year, Day 216. When I moved to Manhattan from The Bronx 27 years ago, I started going to Astor Haircutters which had been open for about 45 years at that point. It was trendy, which I usually don't care about, but also inexpensive, not fancy and big enough so I almost never had to wait. In 27 years maybe once or twice I had to wait about 10 minutes to get my hair cut. When quarantine restrictions were eased, they were one of the first places to open up with masks, social distancing, plastic sheets between chairs. It wasn't enough. A few weeks ago they announced they would close by about Thanksgiving. The business just disappeared. I just went there to get one final cut and spoke to a few staff. My barber had already made plans to get a job at another place and she had one foot out the door. She didn't think there would be any chance the decision would be reversed. When I asked the cashier if business had picked up since the announcement he said "a little" but it sounded very unconvincing. I pointed out to one of the owners that after COVID is gone there will be a lot of empty storefronts and opportunities for a resurrection. He said "we'll see" but as unenthusiastic as the cashier. I recently talked about places that were fighting to stay alive. This place had given up, in spite of the publicity and a

GoFundMe site. I hope things change either now or after COVID. (By the way, I will eventually post about the election but it's too raw a nerve right now. Maybe by Friday.) temp today 98.3

Journal of the Plague Year, Day 217. Yesterday I described the upcoming closing of Astor Hair Cutters. The atmosphere of defeat was overwhelming and upsetting. After I got my haircut and left I recognized that feeling. It was the same feeling I got when St. Vincent's hospital closed. I started working there in 2003 but within a few years the financial problems became overwhelming. One scheme after another was proposed and people were hopeful that the hospital would be saved. When Mount Sinai looked like it would bail us out everyone was joyous. When Sinai changed its mind and withdrew its offer everyone was devastated and everyone completely gave up. Just like the staff at Astor Hair Cutters. Not just logically but emotionally we were drained at the back and forth of imminent disaster. The only good thing that came out of it was that the next job I got was excellent, at least for a while. Also I discovered that the chairman of the Medicine department, my boss, had absolutely excellent brandy and whiskey hidden in his desk draw and we sat, drank, and finished off a few leftover bottles of the best liquor I'd ever had. I don't know how many small businesses in NYC are facing similar financial and emotional defeat at the hands of COVID. I think many will survive, some will be resurrected after this is over, and many new business will spring up. I just hope we don't forget the small places that didn't survive when the good times return in the future, which I'm pretty sure they will. I'll write about what the good times might look like in a future post. temp today. 98.2

Journal of the Plague Year, Day 218. The election still hangs in the balance, although T**** being out looks more likely. But in terms of facing COVID, the public has the same exact options it had in March. Wash hands/sanitize, masks, social distancing, quarantine (both publicly and with businesses). The more we do this as a country the more will survive.

The less we do it more will die, tens or maybe even hundreds of thousands needlessly. If T**** loses, or if he is re-elected and changes his strategy, or if B**** can convince or compel people to do these things will save lives. If T**** is re-elected and keeps his same positions, or if B**** can't convince or compel compliance more will die. And it will stay like that until a vaccine is available which is safe, effective, and widely accepted by the public. It would be nice if we had more options, but we don't. These are the realistic medical options we have and these are the political leaders we have. temp today 98.7 (PS-There is a video on Youtube of "T**** singing Bohemian Rhapsody". It's a very light satire on T**** but funny.)

Journal of the Plague Year, Day 221, Monday November 9. Yesterday when going over the Orchard street for dinner I took a different route. I walked along 14th street from 8th avenue to avenue B at about 4PM. Most weekends I stay south of 14th since uptown recreation (theater, opera, museums, etc) are closed or restricted. From 8th to about 1st avenues there is no parking in the curbside traffic lane, so there are no restaurant/bar enclosures either. From about 1st to B there is both parking and a scattering of curbside enclosures. Coming down B to the downtown streets (Hudson, Bleecker, Orchard, and Mulberry) the dining areas increased a lot. On 14th there were also a bunch of boarded up stores. I couldn't tell if they were vandalized/looted, closed for good, or just being careful. Some of the large stores, especially big chain pharmacies, were had boarded windows but were open for business with their main doors open. Also, for some reason, there were lines of 5-10 people outside two City MD urgent care storefronts. Were they there for flu shots, COVID tests, or what? Temp today 99.0.

Journal of the Plague Year, Day 222. During my walk yesterday afternoon I came across more closed stores and they brought back memories. Right on Perry Street, Kaas glass ware is closing after 18 years. They sold glass items and decoupage, whatever that includes. I never shopped there but now I still feel bad they're closing. They did leave open the possibility of re-locating to another store after the quarantine is over. On avenue A Alphabets is closing. They sold funny greeting cards and chochkas of various types. I bought from there when I needed funny cards or joke gifts. They've had several other stores over the years, so maybe they will re-open later. The Double Down saloon is a dive bar also on A. The NYC Burning Man community used to have weekly happy hours there before moving to Lucky on avenue B (between 10th and 11th). It had a grungy ambience, pool table, back yard and graffiti covered bathroom as required of dive bars. Also cheap drinks. These were all small places that won't make the front pages of any paper. But they also gave NYC a little of it's diversity and character. Something will replace them. We'll see what. temp today. 98.1

Journal of the Plague Year, Day 223. I was going to write about my trip to Arthur Avenue, where I grew up, but since this is Veteran's Day I thought I would write about my dad Stanley instead. He was a WWII Vet and always proud that he served in Africa and Italy. My uncle Jim, a WWII Vet and career army man said my dad was in trouble more than in combat, but that didn't change the fact that he was proud of his service. Growing up in the Bronx he used the VA Hospital on Kingsbridge road for all of his medical care up to including his death from lung cancer (a two pack a day smoker). The care he got there was always good and very comprehensive, which is what most VA hospitals, including the ones I've worked in, are like. He is buried out in Calverton VA cemetery. Thinking about COVID, I realized that I haven't noticed any articles in the medical journals about COVID at VA hospitals. Maybe they were there and I didn't notice since I'm concentrating on nursing homes and assisted livings. In spite of it's bad reputation with the general public, the VA system is one of the, if not the, best systems in the country. It is also a model for a single payer system, at least if it can avoid privatization that is being pushed to take it over. I'll take a closer look at the medical journals and see if COVID at VA hospitals is being reported. Meanwhile, remember veterans. temp today 97.4

Journal of the Plague Year, Day 224. This Monday I went up to Arthur Avenue in the Bronx, where I grew up. It is filled with restaurants, specialty food stores , and an indoor market. It looks entirely Italian even though almost all the Italian Americans moved out and the local resident are mostly Puerto Rican, Albanian, and Mexican. Since it was midday on a work day the neighborhood was fairly quiet and half empty. On the weekend the area is packed with tourists, foodies, shoppers and neighborhood residents, or at least is usually is. But signs of COVID were presents since most of the restaurants and bars had sidewalk shelters. They were empty but there were an awful lot of them, so they must be filled up sometime as much as the downtown streets I've been writing about in these posts. Many of these places are family owned so I think they are as determined to keep going like all the places downtown.

If Arthur Avenue can survive the fifty years of demographic changes that have swept over The Bronx, it should be able to survive this plague. I hope. The mozzarella up there is delicious. temp today 97.6

Journal of the Plague Year, Day 225. I wanted to end on a positive note. This week we had another set of tests on our residents at the ALF. About half of the residents took the test and every one was negative. The staff continues to be tested weekly and we also were entirely negative. Not only does this indicate good policies at the facility, but it means that residents who visit with families and staff are all following safety guidelines when they are outside. I don't know how long this can last, but we have new weapons. We now have the 15 minute Abbott test so we can identify someone who is positive quickly and isolate and contact trace immediately. The rates of cases and deaths are increasing all over the country, including NYC, so I don't know if it will hit us before a vaccine becomes available, but for now our luck is holding out. temp today 98.3

Journal of the Plague Year, Day 228, Monday November 16. I've mentioned before that I like to scoop the mainstream media whenever possible. On Nov 9 I described walking across 14th street on a Sunday afternoon and seeing lines of people in front of two City MD urgent care storefronts. Yesterday on the news City MD announced that it was closing 90 minutes early at all locations due to too much business. If business was so good this would seem to be the time to stay open. But they also explained that the staff at these places were just getting worn out. The time a doc or nurse spend with a patient, giving a COVID test like this case, or doing anything else, is just part of the necessary duties. There is always paperwork and follow-up of some type. I've never worked at one of these storefront places, usually referred to as "Doc In The Box" by the more cynical or jealous members of the medical community, but if they say they're getting burnt out I'm sure they aren't exaggerating. And who knows how frantic or stressed out the patients are who are coming there on a Sunday afternoon at 5. So, Facers, keep reading these posts for breaking news before the breaking news. And if you're one of the mainstream media people reading these and taking my lead, glad to help. temp today 98.6

Journal of the Plague Year, Day 229. The quarantine has put a lot of pressure on the ALF residents where I work. One result is deconditioning. Normally, residents are in and out of their rooms all day, going to meals, activities, leaving the building, going for their medications and generally moving around. At least most of them. But with the quarantine many of them are spending a lot of time sitting in their room all day. Our response is to make occupational and physical therapy as accessible as possible. We have a private rehab group that comes in for homecare OT/PT for many of our residents. At any time there are about 25% of our residents getting OT or PT or both. I don't know if this will keep them fit or conditioned, or decrease falls, or improve mental status by keeping them active. But we are doing as much as we can do and we'll figure it out later if it really helped, or maybe someone else in the medical literature can figure this out. In any case, we're doing the best we can. temp today 98.3

Journal of the Plague Year, Day 230. Yesterday I described how the residents at my ALF are deteriorating physically due to the virus and all the steps to stop it. Today I'll describe the mental deterioration. Before the virus hit, many of my patients had histories of mental health problems of various degrees. sometimes it was mild depression in the distant past, sometimes active depression and/or anxiety with current medications, and sometimes bi-polar or chronic schizophrenia histories. There were days when every patient I saw for medical problems had one of these mental health problems also. The virus has made it worse. Being cooped up in their apartments just brooding, watching (sometimes depressing) TV, or starring at the walls was making many people's depression or anxiety worse. The relaxation of social interaction, common meals, group activities, walks out in the neighborhood or Central Park which is across the street, exercise, family get togethers, etc all helped to minimize symptoms. But they have been minimized or eliminated since March. 8 months of this can drive anyone up the wall. Now there is a little hope. Some of the restrictions are slowly being lifted. Two psychologists have returned and have started to see patients on-site, person to person, which seems much more effective and humane than over Zoom. One specializes in dementia related mental problems and one uses talk therapy. Both of these should help a lot. We are also recruiting for a psychiatrist who can help with medication management a lot better than I can. I hope the worst is over and I hope another lock-down isn't ordered as our COVID tests slowly creep upward. We'll see. temp today 97.9

Journal of the Plague Year, Day 231. After discussing what we have done at my ALF to improve physical and mental health, there is still more. We are trying to increase activities that improve the quality of life at the facility. Our activity room is closed but in the library we are having small groups (5 people max) twice a day for current events discussions, exercise, yoga, and of course bingo. These small groups aren't always filled, so some people are settling into hermit mode and don't come out for any activity. Our lobby is where a half dozen or so people hang out all day. The piano from the activity room is being moved into the lobby and there are several residents who can play it, along with student volunteers and others. Our hair dresser is set to resume sessions soon and that always is a good draw for getting people out of their rooms to socialize. There is a new program of college students who have video/Zoom discussions with residents on a variety of topics, or just to pass the time and provide remote socialization. Unfortunately, one active COVID case will put all of these activities on hold, but for now we are expanding them and hoping more people will get involved. When full, our facility has 127 residents so getting them involved 5 at a time requires a lot of patience. But, there has to be more than providing physical therapy, psychotherapy and cable TV. temp today 98.5

Journal of the Plague Year, Day 232. For almost 20 years at the ALF where I work, residents and staff got flu shots every year with the same approach. One day in flu season, Nov or Dec, community health nurses brought vials of flu vaccine and gave shots to everyone who wanted it. There were usually a few stragglers who were sick on vaccine day, or not in the building, or just didn't want it. Sinai nurses would leave a vial of vaccine with the facility nurses so we could treat these stragglers. This year Sinai was short, so they didn't leave any extra vaccine with us. Today, one resident said he changed his mind and now wanted a shot. We didn't have a supply, and when we contacted the pharmacy we use they said they didn't have any either. They said there was a national shortage. Maybe some of the CityMD storefronts with long lines might have supplies someplace, but I'm not sure. In the words of Sonny, a character in A Bronx Tale, "Youse didn't want a flu shot, well now youse CAN'T GET a flu shot" (see the bar fight scene in the movie). We have to go hunting for someplace that has an extra dose or two. I don't know what this predicts for the coming months when flu season really kicks in. Either it will be much worse on top of COVID cases, or maybe isolation precautions for COVID will make some flu shots less needed. We'll see. temp today 98.5

Journal of the Plague Year, Day 235, Monday November 23. When walking around downtown, I try to draw some lessons about COVID based on my observations. But it's sometimes unclear. This Saturday the doorman of my co-op who drives in from Flushing said the roads were empty and the 45 minute drive only took 20 minutes. Why were the roads empty? Yesterday when going out of my apartment for breakfast at about 10 AM and then dinner at about 5, I noticed something strange. The restaurants were half empty, even those normally packed. breakfast and brunch places on Hudson were half empty instead of people waiting to be seated. On Bleecker and Orchard streets many places were also half empty. On Mulberry, out of 15-20 places two were packed and all the others were almost empty. I don't know if it was the weather, people worried about our COVID numbers rising, people fasting before Thanksgiving feasts, sunspots, or whatever. Maybe my doorman's power of suggestion made be a little more subjective in my observations. Whatever, this is an epidemic with a lot of strange permutations that I'm still trying to figure out. NEWS FLASH-Astor Haircutters will not be closing. Some investors came up with cash to keep them open for the foreseeable future. If true, great news in our battle for normalcy. temp today 98.5

Journal of the Plague Year, Day 236. I've bragged about getting info out faster than the mainstream press and so let me brag a little more. On Nov 5 I mentioned that Astor Hair Cutters was closing, and late last night I mentioned that they had been saved by an investor. Today's NY Daily News, 12 hours after my post, had a front page story on Astor and gave the details of how this family run place was being taken over by investors and will stay open. On Nov 20 I mentioned how we were running short of flu vaccine. Today's Times had an article about a flu vaccine shortage in Italy. I wouldn't be surprised if there was another one soon on flu vaccine shortages in the

US, like I described. Getting stuff out faster than the mainstream is a lot of fun. Makes me feel like what I'm doing is worth it. And that's not counting all the posts I've done on topics that the media didn't pick up. OK, eventually I will say something stupid and the mainstream will come up with a real piece of journalism which makes me look dumb. But, that's the risk you take, like being the first to call an election. There's always a risk of mistakes. In the middle of this life threatening epidemic, if inaccurate posts are the worst mistakes I make, I will be very happy. temp today. 98.6

Journal of the Plague Year, Day 237. There is a lot of news about COVID both good and bad. To end this week on a good note I'll report on a little unofficial unscientific survey I did recently (I'm taking a vacation from posts until Monday Nov 30). A few months ago while sitting and having dinner at various restaurants, I counted the number of people walking by who were wearing masks. About 2/3 had masks and about 1/3 didn't. I repeated this survey last week. While having dinner on Hudson, Orchard, and Mulberry streets at about 5-6 PM on either Friday or Sunday, I counted people with masks. I counted masks under the nose as close enough to be ok, even though technically it isn't, but people wearing masks under their chins were counted as maskless. These were people walking by and not those sitting and eating or drinking. Out of 374 people counted, 320 had masks on and 54 didn't. This worked out to about 14% maskless compared to about 30% a few months ago. 374 is a small number as surveys of this type go, but if this is anywhere near accurate then people are being more careful on the streets. I'm not sure why city wide numbers are going up, but it doesn't appear to be the fault of people walking around, at least not in lower Manhattan. In lower Staten Island the numbers might be different. I'd like to see some government or health care organization repeat this survey around the city to see if street wear could account for the recent increased cases. Something must be doing it, and this is just one of many possibilities. temp today 98.8

Journal of the Plague Year, Day 242, Monday November 30. To keep a somewhat upbeat mood, like last Wednesday, let's go back to the subways. When this started the subways were empty. As they filled up over the months they were also told to wear masks or risk a $50 fine. As the rush hour gets more crowded and a typical car can have 20-30 passengers almost everyone is wearing a mask, and wearing it properly. At the start there were always a handful of people who weren't wearing masks. Now in a fairly full car there might be one or two people either not wearing a mask or wearing it under their chins, so they can flip it up over their nose and mouth quickly if a cop comes. The overall response is much better. A few problems. The Times Square station is still fairly empty so office workers and tourists are still missing. Also the population of subway riders is overwhelmingly minority. I can't remember back to last December so I'm not sure if Times Square, or the ethnic makeup of riders is the way I think it was, but to the best of my recollection that's the way it was. When Times Square fills up or the white folks come back to the subways then those will be even better signs that the city is coming back. Let's hope so. temp today 99.1

Journal of the Plague Year, Day 243. I wrote yesterday about how crowds on the subway described the city, and how the empty Times Square station indicated that the Times Square area above ground was empty. The tourists were gone and the offices were empty. In today's New York Times there was a very long article about how Times Square is empty because all the tourists are gone. I don't know how the Times was able to read my post last night and write such a long article today, but somehow they did. They didn't talk about the office workers. Just one block East of times Square is 6th avenue ("Avenue of the Americas" for the tourists) with is lined with office buildings and normally has big crowds of office workers streaming into the subway stations. Maybe they'll write about that tomorrow. I subscribe to the Times and I'm glad to help them out by feeding information. But remember you Facers who are reading these posts, you'll read it here first. temp today 98.4

Journal of the Plague Year, Day 244. I've started to use another way of monitoring the city during this epidemic. I've noticed that during the day there are a lot more yellow taxis around in the city. I didn't pay attention to this before the pandemic. Taxis were either there or not. Yellow cabs were having a bad time before this all started with competition from on demand services like Uber and Lyft. There were bankruptcies and even suicides. Things have to be worse now. I've mentioned that when coming back from dinner on a typical Sunday night from Orchard or Mulberry street I had problems finding a cab. They weren't coming out because business was so bad, and in midtown (another Times Square reference) it was non-existent. Are the taxis during the daytime finding work? The first few days I started observing more closely I noticed 13 empty cabs and 4 occupied ones on Hudson street and Lower Seventh avenue which is my route going to and coming from the subway when going to work. I'll try to pay attention to this more in the future and report it here. I don't know if the total number will change or the ratio of empty to occupied cabs. We'll see. temp today 98.2

Journal of the Plague Year, Day 245. Another NY Times article about subways both adding to and catching up with what was poster here in April or May. Today's times article looked at the subway stations out in the boroughs instead of Manhattan. It takes a lot for the Times to venture out to the rest of the city but I guess the pandemic did it. They mentioned how more people are using those stations because they are essential workers who can't work remotely. They have low paying jobs and must get to work to provide essential services but also because they can't miss a paycheck. They mention in passing that midtown Manhattan subway traffic is still way down because those workers have higher paying jobs that can be done remotely. The Times is being diplomatic when they refer to low payed essential workers and well payed remote office workers. This really is a case of minority members vs white folks in terms of who is hurt most. If you look at the pictures in the article you could probably figure that the divide is as racial as it is economic or geographic. This might be one of the reasons why mortality rates in minority communities are higher than white areas. In any case, that's the situation we have now, for the time being. This will come up as an important topic when decisions have to be made as to which communities get vaccines first. temp today 98.6

Journal of the Plague Year, Day 246. A little bit of bad news and a lot of good news. I've reported, I think, that the ALF where I work has had a few months without any staff member or resident testing positive for COVID. This week we got a positive COVID test on one of our staff members. We think it might have been a false positive, but there's no way of knowing for sure, so we have to treat it like a real positive. She had a positive nasal swab test on one day and a negative one a week later. We're not sure COVID can actually clear in a week, so that's why we think it might be a false negative.

According to state DOH rules, we now have to go on lock-down for 28 days without visits at the facility. But, there is good news. I was wrong about being clean for a few months. We have been clean for SIX months. In 6 months we have had no resident with a positive test. About half the residents volunteered for tests, all negative. Numerous patients have gone out to the ER or doctor visits and all have been negative. The entire staff gets tested every week and they have been all negative for all six months. So even if this recent case is really positive it is still only one person out of a hundred over six months. I think that's a really good figure. Let's hope it continues until a vaccine becomes available. temp today 97.9

Journal of the Plague Year, Day 249, Monday December 7. A date which will live in infamy even more than November 8, 2016. Last Friday I bragged a little about our relatively good record at the ALF where I work. I forgot to give credit to one possible source of the good news, the

New York State Department of Health. After an initial disaster in the nursing homes the DOH tried to make up for it by countless severe regulations for all long term care facilities, both nursing homes and some assisted living facilities. Just like the countless contradictory pronouncements from the mayor and governor have driven business owners crazy, these DOH regs have sometimes been pretty hard to take. We always complied, eventually, but not without costs. Families cut off from their loved ones usually understood the need, but sometimes they didn't and, I believe, complained to our own facility ombudsman and even to the DOH itself. It's impossible to figure out which of these countless regs had a beneficial effect and which were overkill, but maybe after this is over someone can go over the data and figure out what worked and what didn't so we can do a better job next time. And there will be a next time. temp today 98.3

Journal of the Plague Year, Day 250. Sometimes light and trivial today. My newspaper thefts have probably stopped. The last weekly Times that disappeared happened months ago. I still leave them in the lobby when I go to work, and they are still there when I come home. On the weekend I'm a little more careful. Since the Sunday times is delivered on two days, half on Saturday and half on Sunday, I come down relatively early in the mornings and take The Times and Daily News to my apartment. Relatively early to me is about 10-11 AM but it's earlier than my Noon wake-up time before this all started. This can change at any time, and if this post jinxes things for tomorrow I'll let you know. Tomorrow, a little more serious: vaccines. temp today 97.9

Journal of the Plague Year, Day 251. Talking about vaccines covers a lot or area, so this might take a few days. First, who to believe as info comes out. Don't believe the internet or FB without double checking. I've seen things on FB that were helpful accurate and came out faster than on the mainstream media. But I've also seen a vast amount of crap. So far the drug companies have been putting out info through their press offices and the media have been putting it out in the most optimistic was possible. What we have to look for are reports from the media that aren't so upbeat, since there will be problems. The FDA is supposed to put out a report soon on the Pfizer vaccine, and eventually the Moderna vaccine. We'll have to try and judge if it's a whitewash or an accurate evaluation. Also look at info from the CDC like the post that I just saw here above my post. Their website is big and going through it might take time to find something clear and simple and not in bureaucratic jargon, but their announcements will also come out in the media and usually in a simpler form. Simple put, be careful what you see in the next few days/weeks. I'll be giving a lot more info here about what to avoid, swine flu history, description of what I'm going to do for myself and my patients. Watch this space. temp today 97.0

Journal of the Plague Year, Day 252. The Pfizer vaccine has tentative approval from an FDA advisory committee. It will probably get complete emergency approval soon. All the news looks good, but let me tell you that when a new medicine comes our, or even an old medicine, it is almost never without problems eventually. This will go to hundreds of thousands of people, and eventually millions. Rare side effects that you wouldn't see in initial safety studies might be seen with millions of patients. Watch for this. Anti-v****** will publicize, exaggerate, or sometimes even make up stories about the vaccine. People normally get other diseases just by coincidence. If a million people took the vaccine on a Monday, that Tuesday morning some who appeared completely healthy will have heart attacks, strokes, brain tumors, tooth aches, autism or terminal flatulence just by pure coincidence. It's just in the numbers. The approval for the vaccine said that the benefits outweigh the possible risk. This is always the case with any medicine and there will be risks and side effects. If the overall benefit is great, given that COVID can kill you, it would be beneficial to take the vaccine unless the harm is really really significant. Don't be freaked out over news, like those two women in England who had severe allergic reactions after the vaccine. And, it's happened before. Tomorrow, swine flu. temp today 98.5

Journal of the Plague Year, Day 253. There have been various viral infections that hit the world over the last decades, several called Swine Flus even though some did not clearly original in pigs In 2009 the H1N1 flu, a combination of typical annual flu and a new strain, hit the US with about 12,000 estimated deaths. In 1976 there was another swine flu which was a little more controversial. It killed a relatively small number of people, possibly fewer than a few hundred, but the vaccine to it (which might account for the small number of deaths) caused Guillaine-Barre syndrome which is a form of post viral paralysis. As many as 500 people got that with about 25 deaths. It was called a fiasco because the vaccine might have caused as much damage as the infection. That's what we know in hindsight. Unfortunately, we don't have hindsight now with COVID. We have, in the US, about 300,000 deaths and an overall mortality rate of about 2%. When the various vaccines come out they could easily have side effects we don't know about yet. At that time, some anti-v****** and anti-maskers will point to the side effects, minimize the deaths (they were old or sick and would die anyway) and claim the entire plague was a conspiracy or hoax to make the drug companies rich, or make doctors rich, or embarrass T****, or whatever. It is very unlikely that vaccine side effects when they occur, and they probably will occur, will produce a mortality greater than 2% or whatever the final rate is. Remember, don't get distracted by the complaints and conspiracies, but keep your eye on the ball. The disease kills, the vaccines help, usually. temp today 98.0

Journal of the Plague Year, Day 256, Monday December 14th. I've done a few posts about the vaccine, but the bottom line is what will I do for myself, my staff, and my patients. It looks like the hospital front line people are getting the vaccine first, which I agree with. Nursing home staff and patients should be second. Assisted living residents and staff, including me, should be next. This is assuming an orderly distribution with sufficient vaccine doses, but we don't know if either assumption is true. Since I don't know what the future brings and don't know what problems can arise, I'm opting for getting the vaccine as soon as possible. As previously mentioned, there is always a chance of unforeseen side effects and problems, but there is also a chance of unforeseen COVID infections and death. I'll let you all know when I get my first shot. temp today 98.0. My first reading after drinking a cold soda was 95.8 which couldn't be right. I waited about 5 minutes and took it again to get 98.0. This is a problem. When I go into work they take my temp at the door and it is always too low, sometimes the thermometer even reads "LO". I have to go down to my office and later have one of the nurses take my temp. The importance of this is that for job sites and eventually indoor dining again, the quick temp on the forehead might not be accurate and someone reading 97 might actually be 100.7 after a few minutes. I don't know how to control for this just yet, but maybe when the weather gets better this will be a moot point. We'll see.

Journal of the Plague Year, Day 257. So let's say we all get our vaccines. Are we done? No, unfortunately. There are still a few things that can cause damage and that we don't have the answers to. First, can people who are immune to COVID from vaccine or infection be carriers and still infect other people? We don't know that for sure. So, those of us who will be immune still need to wear our masks until this is answered. Second, does a person's immunity change or last forever, like measles or for a few years, like pneumonia, or only a year like flu. We may need to do this whole vaccine routine yearly if our immunity is weak. That's why the CDC, from a memo I've seen, recommend people who have had the disease and should be immune should STILL get the vaccine. This is based on the possible unreliability of a person's immune system. At least from what we know now. Third, will the virus mutate? There are several strains of the virus now, some which travel quickly, after only being around for a year. Vaccine researchers say these mutations are minor and the different strains should all be susceptible to the vaccines. But, what if the next mutations aren't so minor? The virus itself must have mutated from some previously existing virus, so a mutation that produces a brand new virus with brand new virulence is not out of the questions. And these are just the three problems I can think up, and I'm not a specialist in this area. More problems might show up later. Let's hope they're all "minor". temp today 98.7

Journal of the Plague Year, Day 258. Oops, forgot a few things yesterday. A few more things we don't know about COVID. Fourth, we don't know if people can get the full infection more than once. A combination of incomplete, or fading away immunity, in combination with subtle changes in the virus might give more than one infection. The disease is only a year old so we might need more time. Fifth, speaking of time, we don't know about long range effects. Lots of influenza and pneumonia infections come and go but don't leave permanent damage to the lungs. Other diseases like emphysema and bronchiectasis, and sometimes tuberculosis can leave permanent damage to the lungs which persists and decreases pulmonary function long after the initial infection is gone. Sixth, COVID produces inflammation and blood clots throughout the body, not just the lungs. What immediate and what long term damage can be done to other organs in the body that we don't know about yet. When more COVID deaths are examined with autopsies we may start to see other damage throughout the body that were asymptomatic, or just missed. OK, enough dark medical stuff, I'll try and find something lighter for tomorrow. temp today 98.6

Journal of the Plague Year, Day 259. Delis, bodegas, and all the other places we get our breakfast coffee and danish/bec sandwiches need a little attention. I don't know if these are only NYC traditions. Years ago there was an exhibit in Grand Central

Station about movies made about NYC like King Kong or others. There was a picture of Holly Golightly, played by Audrey Hepburn, standing outside Tiffaney's jewelry store in the movie Breakfast at Tiffaney's. Holly had a coffee in one hand and a danish in the other and the caption said "Holley Golightly having "breakfast" in front of Tiffaney's" Quotes around breakfast?! A coffee and danish, as far as I'm concerned is breakfast , not "breakfast" in NYC. Was this caption writer from Connecticut or Iowa or what? For the next few posts I'll be talking about this NYC institution (delis, not Tiffaney's). A lot light topic than vaccines and death rates. temp today 98.1

Journal of the Plague Year, Day 260. I had been planning to write about the delis/bodegas that I use for breakfast in my neighborhood and near work. What finally pushed me was the sudden closing of a small Korean (I think) deli a week ago. One victim of COVID, but there are many others fighting COVID and desperately trying to survive. A few things in common: determination and immigrants. Of the places I have gone, three are run by Dominicans (DR not nuns), two by Egyptians (Copts I think), one by Asian Indians (a Dunkin Donuts) and the recently closed Korean place. Only one place, a Starbucks I rarely go to, is run by presumably American born millenials. Several of these places are run by families. This is what first generation entry level immigration does for the US. One daughter is working in the deli while finishing her bachelor's degree in engineering. Engineering!

Similar attempts at upward mobility exist in a lot of the immigrant families of low income workers in the nursing homes and assisted living facilities I've worked in. Widescale limiting of immigration will hurt all these industries, not to mention the highly trained foreigners flooding into Silicon Valley, and maybe even leave us without our morning coffee and danish! I hope this is reversed quickly. And, all these people seem determined to keep their businesses open in spite of COVID. Longer hours, smaller staffs and just plain hard work. And always the risk of bankruptcy and failure in spite of all the work. I hope they all survive until the plague is over. temp today 98.2

Journal of the Plague Year, Day 263, Monday December 21. I mentioned the delis/bodegas that I have been using since before the epidemic. There is something I noticed and I am asking other Facers, especially in the city, to address this. The three Dominican bodegas I go to all do the same thing. They wrap the coffee in a paper bag, put it in a larger paper or plastic bag, and then put the danish or bec sandwich in the same bag. One bag holds everything. When I walk I can carry everything in one hand and my other is completely free. The other places, korean, egyptian, Dunkin and Starbucks, especially Starbucks put all the food in one bag and the coffee separately. It is easier to drink the coffee while walking (and showing off the Starbucks logo in the process) but you have to use both hands to carry. Is this observation universal? If you go to latino bodegas and get coffee and danish/bec see if they put everything in one bag without prompting. If you go to any other breakfast place, especially Dunkin or Starbucks, see if they always put the coffee separately. This isn't the most important question we have to answer right now, and I can't come up with a way to link this to COVID, but I need a few lighter posts before Christmas so we don't all go into the holiday on a down note. There will be plenty of time for that later. temp

Journal of the Plague Year, Day 264. I thought I noticed another upbeat post I could do to give us an upbeat Christmas season. This time of the year, the assisted living facility where I work gets a lot of Christmas gifts. Families, friends, colleagues and co-workers bring in food, baked goods, candies, countless chocolates, an occasional bottle of booze and, when we're lucky, coquito. I thought that this year the bounty of gifts were significantly more than previous years. I figured this was a reaction to the stress from COVID. One of the administrators thought our annual Christmas haul was the same as always but it was compressed over the last few days instead of the last few weeks, and so appeared more significant. I'm unconvinced and will ask for a second opinion among other staff members. Meanwhile, I will persist in my belief (or perhaps delusion) that this year produced a bumper crop of gifts, implying a bumper crop of appreciation for what we do under the present difficult circumstances. temp today 98.5

Journal of the Plague Year, Day 265. A melancholy note today. Why do I put my temperature in these posts? Partly it's so Facers reading this have a little more insight into the day to day monitoring we have to do. Fortunately, so far, no major illness or drama has been linked to these temps. But I got the idea originally from Florent. Florent was a restaurant in the Meatpacking district which was one of the first (along with Hogs and Heffers) that started to change the area from meatpacking plants and trans prostitutes into a gentrified playground for the beautiful people. Florent Morellet, the owner, was a gay may who eventually tested positive for HIV. On the board that announced the daily specials, Florent posted his T-cell numbers from his most recent test, as a rough correlate of the seriousness of his active infection. There was nothing that could be done with this number even by a physician like me. It was just a heartfelt sharing of a very personal aspect of Florent's life. My daily temps are a feint shadow of what he did, but it's the same idea. It helps us all identify with what the writer, me, is going through. It's not that significant or dramatic, so far, just a minor episode of sharing.

By the way, the restaurant was a great place. Open 24 hours, young people, old people, neighborhood people, bridge and tunnel people, families with kids, trans street walkers, good inexpensive French bistro food. Very hip environment. After theater, opera, parties, etc, this was the late night place to go. The same gentrification the Florent helped start eventually killed it with a dramatic increase in rent. I personally think he could easily have raised prices for his loyal customers, but after twenty years it just might have been time for him to move on. He now lives in Brooklyn, I believe, and a recent interview indicated he might be looking into something in the hospitality field, maybe a bar and not a restaurant. He also is an artist specializing in fantasy maps, which I think is pretty unique. There is a film

"Florent, Queen of the Meat Market" somewhere on the internet. And if you ever saw him dressed up as Marie Antoinette on Bastille Day you know that Queen is the proper adjective. But now L'Avventura est fini (the same notice he had on the restaurant board after the death of director Michelangelo Antonioni). Long post today but I'll be resting until Monday December 28th. temp today 98.3

Journal of the Plague Year, Day 270, Monday December 28. I thought that once the epidemic is all over NYC would start to rebound and I could do a post on resilience and rebuilding the city. I was wrong. Rebounding has already started but I didn't really notice it until today. Coming back from work I past the corner store where Two Boots pizza used to be on the corner of Greenwich avenue and seventh avenue. In tremendous red letters there was a new announcement of Zazzy's Pizza. Zazzy's Pizza?! I never heard of it, and what was it doing moving into this spot? It's actually a traditional and also vegan, or at least vegetarian pizza place with a store on Orchard street. I must have passed it many times. Now it was expanding to the West side in the middle of this plague. I started to think of the other places. There are several new clothing stores on Bleecker just opening or about to open. Cafe Dante's branch on Hudson opened in the middle of the pandemic, and is going strong. Many restaurants, though far from all, are still packing in sidewalk business even after indoor dining was banned again. I assume many new businesses know they won't make money to begin with, so having enough cash to carry them at the start-up before they hopefully take off. That dead period might as well come in the middle of all this as well as any other time, especially if they could make a deal on the rent for one of the countless empty storefronts. These small new shoots are popping up all over. The rebound has started. How strong will it be? Nobody knows yet, but keep your eyes open. It's here. temp today 98.1

Journal of the Plague Year, Day 271. (a little late) Yesterday I posted about stuff happening in my neighborhood indicating resilience. At the alf where I work there are also some signs of this. A newsletter put together by residents with a little help from staff has resurfaced. In the past it was done all by residents, but this is a start. Most of the articles were written by staff people but there were a few poems written by residents and a holiday wish from the president of the resident committee which represent the wishes, complaints, activities and suggestions from the residents. Tomorrow there will be a New Year's Eve party, though in the afternoon, on New Year's Eve Eve and with faux cocktails (mocktails) along with some gift giving. The lobby is still filled with residents during the day, although filled with appropriate social distancing. Sometimes there is a musical piece by one of our retired jazz musicians. These are small steps back to normalcy, and they can all disappear if the numbers get worse or if the DOH comes down with new restrictions. But, this is the best we have now, and we are still being very cautious. As one of our residents wrote in the newsletter "It's not a big task, just wear your mask!" temp today 97.9

Journal of the Plague Year, Day 272. (very late today, is that red wine with dinner getting stronger or am I getting more feeble/tired?). There have been reports that there are many members of minority communities who are skeptical about taking the COVID vaccine. Because of medical scandals in the past, and lots of inequality in the delivery of services right now, many minority members don't trust the health care system. But, there is one aspect of the health care system that will actually benefit minority members more than the general population. Many nursing homes and assisted living facilities have many minority workers who are essential but underpaid. In the alf where I work, about 90% of the staff are minorities. This might even be true if you look at the total workforce in hospitals. All of these places, hospitals, nursing homes and alfs, are getting the first shot at the COVID vaccines. So the staff members, including a disproportionate number of people of color, will actually be among the first to get access to a medical service instead of being among the last. This is truly a case of "the last shall be first..." but only if people accept the vaccine. Refusing it doesn't correct any of past or present abuses by the healthcare system, but accepting it gives one of the few cases where being a low paid worker actually helps, although it is entirely accidental. temp today 98.3

Journal of the Plague Years, Day 277, Monday January 4. Yes, the plague years, not just one year. Exactly one month ago, the NY Times wrote an article about the taxi industry in London and how many taxi drivers can't make a living because of the COVID pandemic ("Field of Broken Dreams", London Taxis Growing Graveyards.) I'm glad it gave Mark Landler, the author, a chance to go to London on the Times dime, but I've been looking at taxis here in NYC. A while back I mentioned that I'm counting the ratio of empty vs filled taxis in NYC. I've only looked in the West Village either during rush hours or dinner time. I actually lost the paperwork and data I was collecting, so let me give you approximate numbers. The ratio of empty to filled taxis ranged from 5 to 1 to 10 to 1. the overwhelming majority of cabs are empty. How can they survive? Before COVID the yellow cab industry was in trouble with Uber/Lyft competition and even taxi driver suicides. When I take a taxi I always ask how business is, and they have always said it is bad and that midtown (23-57 street) is even worse. I don't know how they can survive except out of shear determination. Good luck to them. Maybe some day the Times can write a follow up article on taxis in NYC, not just London. temp today 98.1

Journal of the Plague Years, Day 278. New York Magazine had a long detailed article about COVID and how it actually could have been an accidental release from a Chinese laboratory. Lots of speculation but not impossible. I didn't even read it, because it's irrelevant at this point. If they accidentally released it when doing research on it (possible) and then tried to minimize the damage (definite) that's not that different from some other countries, including us, at the start. We minimized the risk and instead of doing what might help (complete national shut down for 6-8 weeks, masks, social distancing) we also minimized it and half the country denied it was even a problem, until it was too late. Some parts of the country even now deny it's a problem whether Staten Island, Brooklyn or Alabama (I pick on Alabama because I don't know how to spell Mississippi). At this point we have to use these incomplete tools as much as possible while the vaccines get distributed and used. We might eventually figure out all the lies and mistakes of the past, but right now it doesn't help us. More on conspiracies tomorrow and vaccines later in the week. temp today 99.2

Journal of the Plague Years, Day 279. Yesterday on the subway there was an elderly guy, wearing a mask, who was handing out a one page flyer with all sorts of anti-COVID paranoia. It was a fraud, no worse than the flu, masks don't work, social distance doesn't work, and imposition of all these measures is a way for the government to impose controls on the people and take away our freedoms! A vast amount of paranoid nonsense. But with what happened today in DC we can see what happens when paranoia gets out of control. T**** won the election in a landslide, the D*** conducted fraud, the election was a fraud, etc etc. Some of the people who believe the election was a fraud also probably believe COVID is a fraud. This is what happens when you let paranoia and lies get out of control. It's a lot easier to unleash craziness for your own purposes than it is to control it once unleashed. Will the anti-COVID, anti-v****** paranoids start carrying guns to protect themselves from the oppressive mask imposing government. Who knows? But if you think that's not going to happen then look at the news a few more times and see what happened today when the fanatics and paranoids took control in DC. And, as any mental health worker can tell you, people suffering from paranoia can sometimes be very dangerous. temp today 98.1

Journal of the Plague Years, Day 280. The last two days, in the middle of yesterday's terrible news, I'm going to try and be upbeat. (my political views are on my front page, I'm not sure what it's called. This page is for COVID stuff, at least for now.) A few days ago I saw a young women walking along Hudson street with a cap that had the slogan "New York or nowhere". That's part of the attitude that is going to make NYC bounce back after this plague is over. After 9/11 in 2001 the population of NYC went up a few hundred thousand. Everyone knew that NYC was the target for every terrorist group in the world, yet people moved in. I think the same happened after hurricane Sandy even though everyone knows that this city of islands is vulnerable to rising oceans. One thing that slows recovery is the high price or rents, and everything else, in NYC. But after the plague there will be a lot of empty storefronts and apartments. The law of supply and demand will still be in effect so if prices come down and demand is high people and businesses will flood in. And, people and businesses will still want to be in NYC. There always are. Everyone knows the term "...if you can make it there you can make it anywhere." I think that it will be just as attractive in the future. We'll see. temp today 98.0

Journal of the Plague Years, Day 281. In spite of the political events of this week (look at the intro FB screen, however you get there) I'm still going to try and be upbeat about the future of NYC. Yesterday I went to the new Moynihan station. It's big, well lit with natural lighting, has bathrooms for men, women, and non-gender specific that are cleaner than some of the hospital operating rooms I've seen, at least for now. A food court area that will be opening in the future. One big project is not enough to re-vitalize a city as big as NYC, but there is a lot more going on. 9/11 attack, Sandy, ridiculous rents and a once a century epidemic have slowed but not stopped the city. After 9/11 it only took a few days for the majority of the city outside lower Manhattan to get moving again. Hudson yards, embankments for surge protection, projected multi-billion dollar improvements of rail lines and tunnels, and whatever the new regime in Washington is likely to provide keep the city moving. According to a TV news report, some neighborhoods have rent decreases from 1 to 25%. There will be a flood of people coming back. Years ago I was speaking to a woman who moved here from Germany, who said that what impressed her about NYC was its efficiency. Efficiency in NYC?! Yes, she pointed out that no matter what happens to the city it seems to just keep going with millions of people flowing into and out of it every day like a river. That reminded me of a metaphor for NYC. In the song "Old man river" the Mississippi is described as just rolling along although the people around it come and go and are forgotten. That's what NYC is like. It just keeps rolling on no matter what. And, I think it will continue to do so for the foreseeable future. How's that for an upbeat ending to a horrible week? temp today 98.6

Journal of the Plague Years, Day 284, Monday January 11. I've talked about what it would take for NYC to bounce back. Lower rents, help from Washington, eventually ending the pandemic, etc. There's one thing I forgot. The determination of native New Yorkers, not business owners, to survive in the city. I mentioned on women with a "New York or nowhere" hat. Yesterday on Christopher street I passed two women, one of whom was gesturing to something she saw on the street and commented to the other "what a great fucking city." I don't know what she was pointing to, or even if she was talking about NYC, but it seemed appropriate. This attitude isn't new. In the 1957 movie "The Sweet Smell of Success" Burt Lancaster and Tony Curtis are coming out of a bar and they notice a drunk being tossed out onto the street. They take this in for a second and Burt turns to Tony and says "I love this dirty town". There are lots of people who hate the city and will leave as soon as possible, others who are so-so and will take what comes, but a core of us are determined to ride this out. I haven't seen a cap that says "This dirty fucking town or nowhere" yet, but I'll keep looking for one. temp today 98.7

Journal of the Plague Years, Day 285. A few weeks ago indoor dining was again banned in NYC. There was a lot of worry among restaurant owners that this would kill more of them. Every once in a while there is another post mentioning that some restaurant is boarded up and might be dead. But, there are still a lot that are staying open in spite of the indoor dining ban. Two days ago I took my usual walk along the streets of lower Manhattan (Hudson, Bleecker, Orchard, Mulberry) at about 4-5 PM. A lot of outdoor sidewalk seating areas were set up but about 50% were not open to serve food. They weren't boarded up, just not up and serving. About 25% were opened and about half filled, and the last 25% were opened and packed with customers. Every seat taken a a few people waiting to be seated. I don't know what distinguishes an empty or half-empty place from a hot thriving place. Food, word of mouth, trendiness, whatever. Maybe if I figure this out I'll be able to open a place some day, after retirement. We'll see. temp today 98.1

Journal of the Plague Years, Day 286. Today I'm going to talk about getting a shoe shine at Penn Station. It doesn't take much to see that talking about a shoe shine doesn't amount to a hill of beans in this crazy world (I love quoting Casablanca). But this is another case of trying, perhaps futilely, to get back to normal. A while back I talked about my haircutting place, Astor Haircutters, being closed because of COVID, and then saved by some local rich guy. It's now open. In Penn Station there was a shoe shine place that I've probably been going to for many years right across from the NJ Transit waiting area. After work at about 4 or 5 I would go there and get a good shoe shine from the 6 or so workers. The last few times I went it was closed, so I thought it was dead. But, there was a cell phone number which I called and the person on the other end said it had been sold to a new owner but was only opened from 9:30 to 3, when it closed for lack of customers. Today I went at about 2 PM. (I make my own hours. It's good to be the doctor. Another movie reference). There were two people instead of 6-7 and one other customer besides myself. Price had gone up from $5 to 8. The two people working there were middle aged Latinos and it looked like they were still getting up to full speed since they were sharing some of the materials/ equipment. But they were working like crazy to do a good job, which they did for me and the construction worker sitting a few chairs away. I hope they survive and I hope the very empty Penn station gets busy. Resuming haircuts and shoeshines is a really, really small step towards normalcy. But right now I'll take what I can get when I can get it, and hope that the big stuff (vaccines) come through soon. We'll see. temp today 98.6

Journal of the Plague Years, Day 287. New Yorkers are trying to get back to normal, as I've described over the last few posts. We are also trying to get back to our obsessions, even when they're not that "normal". For example, our obsessions with trendy foods. Magnolia bakery is in my neighborhood and is known for it's cupcakes. After appearing on a few TV shows, SNL and I think Sex in the City, it developed a fanatical following. Before the plague there were often long lines in front of it. I just noticed, that when I come home at around 5-6 PM there are lines there again. Only a few in the store and maybe a half dozen at most outside, but still lines in 30-40 degree weather. For cupcakes and delicious layer cakes. On Prince street, 27 Prince to be exact, there is Prince Street Pizza. It used to be the site of Ray's Pizza which was famous for the quality of it's food but also for the legal fight over the use of it's name. Ray's is gone but Prince has a following. They also had a very well publicized legal fight over the right to make, and advertise, a very spicey pepperoni slice. I don't know how good it is, but when I pass Prince street on my Sunday night walks over to Orchard street, there is always a long line in front of it. The last few weeks there have been 30-40 people on line at 4-5 PM Sunday. 30-40 for a slice of pizza! When the weather is good there is often a line of a dozen or so in front of Joe's Pizza on Carmine street. I don't know how may on line are local natives, bridge and tunnel people, or tourists (if there are any tourists around), but these ridiculous lines are a sure sign of the return of our normal level of insanity when it comes to food. Now if I can only figure out when these lines are shorter, I can join in this insanity. Hmm...pizza! temp today. 98.5

Journal of the Plague Years, Day 288. And now...vaccines. There is a lot in the mass media about what is happening with vaccines. Some major hospitals are running out ahead of schedule. Some states are given a short count of doses delivered by the feds. The public is sometimes having difficulty making appointments at some of the vaccination venters, and other times there are no problems. There is so much variability that it's hard to describe it all. I will try to describe what is happening at my level, in the trenches at a facility that is actually doing the vaccinations. New week 1/3 the staff, including myself, will be getting it and all the residents who want it. There is paperwork that is being filled out now with medical history and written permission to get the shot. Only 1/3 are getting it so that if there are a lot of side effects and people call in sick the facility won't be short staffed the next day. Will there be problems? We'll see. temp today 98.4

Journal of the Plague Years, Day 292, Tuesday Jan 19th. Tomorrow I should get my vaccine. What can go wrong and what can go right? First, some history. In 1947 several cases of smallpox were detected in NYC. The NYC Health Commissioner Israel Weinstein started a major vaccination program to inoculate all NYC. Public health workers started thc program, they borrowed vaccines from all over, police and fire departments helped out and eventually US military helped. In about a month 4-6 million New Yorkers were vaccinated (this is all from a fast internet search). The spread was stopped at about a dozen cases and a few deaths, and many years later using similar vaccination programs, smallpox was eliminated from the earth. What did they have that we don't? We don't have a large supply of vaccine for COVID. There is very little public health structure now, so vaccinations are divided between pharmacies (CVS and Walgrens), hospitals, county health departments, special sites opening up, etc. There was one person,

Weinstein, in control, not different Health Commissioners, a Mayor, a Governor, someone or another in the Federal system, etc. There was case tracing for the few cases that were first detected. And, the public didn't view smallpox as a hoax and resist vaccination. So, we have a lot of problems and a brand new virus, COVID19, not to mention the new mutations that are appearing. We'll see how this plays out. temp today 98.8

Journal of the Plague Years, Day 293. Got my first Pfizer COVID vaccine shot today, and I feel TERRIBLE! My arm is swollen like it will drop off, I have a temp and shaking chills. I feel like I'm going to DIE!... OK, only kidding. I feel fine, and this is the easiest vaccine I've ever taken. The needle was smaller than the the annual flu vaccine (0.3cc vs 0.5cc) and I really couldn't even feel it when they stuck me. There were 8 people sent from CVS to administer the vaccine and they were really efficient. This same team had done a lot of vaccinations at a lot of places and it was like an assembly line. I sat around for 15 minutes under observation, and they really played it by the book. Exactly 15 minutes! We do this again for the booster dose in 21 days, exactly. More details tomorrow. temp today 98.3

Journal of the Plague Years, Day 294. Yesterday I described how efficient the CVS staff was at vaccinations. The efficiency was similar to what public health nurses from years ago exhibited before public health systems were allowed to deteriorate. But, I digress. Here's the results from my facility. We have about 101 residents living in the building now and about 84 got the vaccine. Another three or so will be getting it once some paperwork is completed. 87 out of 101 is pretty good. The staff was scheduled to have one third of its 100 people but about 38 got it. In 21 days they will return to give boosters for yesterdays recipients and more vaccines for the remaining people who need it. The CVS staff said that the supply of vaccine has been put aside and is not being used up for others. I hope so. In three weeks we'll see how many of the remaining staff actually get the vaccine, since many appear hesitant. Any problems that popped up will be posted tomorrow once I gather all the hard data and soft gossip. temp today 98.7

Journal of the Plague Years, Day 295. So, after all the worries about the vaccine, what negative effects did we get? At least four employees were sick, some with aches, chills and low temperatures. A few called in sick for one or two days, but all are ok now. One patient thinks he got sick and very weak from the vaccine, but we can't be sure that's what actually did it. Some staff and patients may have gotten sick that I don't know about, but so far it looks like these are the only problems. Our staff and patients talk among themselves, so it's unclear if these few cases will scare other people off getting the vaccine. We'll see in 3 weeks. In general, most people who had a problem have a little tenderness at the injection site, but that's no worse than our annual flu shots. Compared to the problems of actually getting COVID, this isn't much. And, the rate of COVID running around the city is still high. More on COVID spread next week, but for now let's end the week on a high note of how the vaccine is finally getting to the people who need it. temp today 98.3

Journal of the Plague Year, Day 298. In the past I've bragged about how the assisted living facility where I work had such good covid statistics. Well, it couldn't last forever. First, the good news. The half of our residents who want covid testing are still 100% negative. But the staff are starting to show positive tests. A few weeks ago, two staffers in the same department tested positive. A week later five staffers, in different departments, tested positive. Some of them had covid cases at home, so conversion wasn't a surprise. Others exposure is unclear. In fact, with five positive in one day, we're not even sure if some of the tests were false positives. But a positive is a positive and we couldn't take a chance. All stayed away or are staying away from work for two weeks. I don't know if any of these were symptomatic or if they were picked up on our weekly random testing. tomorrow-how this happened. temp today 98.4

Journal of the Plague Year, Day 299. Before I explain how covid seeped into my facility, one more piece of bad news. None of our residents tested positive starting in July and ending this weekend. The first resident in so many months tested positive. He had a respiratory illness with symptoms that had been building for a few days, unresponsive to antibiotics, and this weekend was sick enough to go into the hospital where he tested positive for covid. Well, a perfect record for 6 months is pretty good, but it's a shame it couldn't keep going. Since he is still in the hospital, I'm not sure how severe or life threatening it will be. How he got it, we don't know. He may have been out of the building one day recently or maybe he came into contact with one of our staff cases. It's hard to know for sure. What we do know is that the floor he is on is on somewhat of a lockdown and receiving increased monitoring. As a matter of fact, since the staff tested positive over the last few weeks, the entire facility is on increased lock down with no group activities at all and no hanging out in the lobby,, even with 6 feet of separation. This might last a week or two if there are no new cases. A few days of bad news, and maybe more tomorrow, is a downer. But, I'm going to try and save the good news, and there is good news, for the end of the week so we can go into the weekend on an up note. At least, that's the plan. temp today 98.8

Journal of the Plague Years, Day 300. So, how did covid seep back into my assisted living facility? It's not too hard to figure out, considering what we already knew about flu transmission, along with common sense. In the past it was shown that if you want to keep influenza out of a nursing home it's more effective to vaccinate the staff than the residents. That's where the common sense comes in, either with flu or covid. Staff come and go in and out of the facility and mingle with lots of people at their homes, with friends, relatives, people in stores, subway/bus riders, etc. They have orders of magnitude more contact with other people than nursing home or assisted living residents who are surrounded by a small circle of friends or staff. It only takes one wrong contact to spread an infectious disease. The spread of covid in the staff isn't only not surprising but it's almost inevitable. temp today 98.5

Journal of the Plague Years, Day 301. In my facility, state regs require that residents are informed whenever a staff member or resident is positive for covid. The staff and resident infections I've posted on recently have been communicated to everyone in the facility. That might account for what happened today. When residents were first given the option to get tested for covid, about half got tested. Today about 84 of about 90 agreed to the test. As the infections keep happening people are paying more attention. That's among the residents, whose average age is in the low 80s. On Feb 10 the next round of vaccines will be administered. Let's see if the rest of the staff, about 60 or so, will follow the residents lead and start taking this seriously, or will they still be too frightened to get their shots. We'll see. temp today 98.3

Journal of the Plague Years, Day 302. To end on a high note, let's talk influenza. Influenza? At the start of this plague there was a worry that the winter would simultaneously hit us with the covid cases along with the flu cases that hit us every year. But, this year the rate of influenza cases is about 1-2% of what it was in previous years at this time (Jan 15 issue of Science magazine, or http://www.health.ny.gov/.../comm.../influenza/surveillance/ . I don't know if this link will work. I get it as a NY Physician from the state Department of Health. Facers reading this, let me know if you could open the link. It shows very dramatically that there is almost no flu, when compared to previous years. There was a slight increase in people taking the flu vaccine, from about 50% to 60% of those who could take it. But that increase is too small to account for the dramatic differences. The only reasonable explanation is that the same methods to control the respiratory disease covid is also controlling the respiratory disease influenza (masks, isolation, social distancing, red wine). For the future, this also shows that maybe these non-vaccine methods can actually be used against all respiratory diseases. It's a very good and unexpected result of this epidemic, a little silver lining in this dark covid cloud. temp today 97.6

Journal of the Plague Years, Day 305. I usually try to post about something low level that the main stream media miss. But today I'll comment on something in the media. The Times reported that many public health experts working for t,he state of NY quit because C**** was being a jerk, overriding their decisions, and making decisions of his own without consulting them. This is very T****-like "I know better than the experts" behavior. C****'s behavior in general isn't a surprise but his involvement in health decisions is new to me. Doing daily press conferences (also very T****-like) don't help if you're making the wrong decisions. This is a new story so more info might come out explaining this internal C**** vs public health experts fight, but now this is what we have. I'll be looking for more. Of course, if he did take control then he has to take responsibility for things that go wrong, like expanding those who could take the vaccine before the vaccine is available. But, like a stopped clock, even C**** can sometimes be correct. I'll try tomorrow to give an example of a controversy where C**** might be right and unfairly criticized. temp today. 98.7

Journal of the Plague Years, Day 306, Tuesday Feb 2 (Happy Groundhog Day!). Leticia James reported (sued?) C**** because he understated nursing home covid deaths. Sorry I don't have inside information on this, but I do have a little experience. When someone gets sick in a nursing home, or in the community, and are sent to the hospital they are then considered hospital patients and not listed as community or nh patients. If they die in the hospital, it is held responsible for the death until proven otherwise. If it was an expected death from whatever illness it is considered a hospital death and the hospital is held accountable. If the death is not easily explained the medical examiner can examine the case, especially if the person was admitted within 24 hours. Whatever is found is put on the record for the hospital and if they screwed up they might be held accountable. So, if the people who got sick in the nursing home and died in the hospital are considered hospital deaths rather than nursing home deaths, I think this is normal procedure before covid ever arrived on the scene. If Leticia James wants to blame C**** and the state DOH for listing as hospital deaths those illnesses that started in the nursing home then this is misclassification not suppression of data and I think there's a big difference. I haven't worked on the wards in a hospital in over 10 years so my memory of this might be rusty, but I think it's true. If you die in the hospital it is a hospital death no matter where you got sick. Facers reading this post with more experience than I have can chime in on this if they like. temp today 98.7

Journal of the Plague Years, Day 307. I'm trying to plan this year's schedule. Not my work, which will go on, but special events. There is a convention of the American Medical Directors Association in March which will be all virtual, like it was last year. But, Burning Man, which normally occurs the last week of August and was cancelled last year, is still up in the air. It's hard to know exactly how bad or how controlled covid will be in August. Burners sent out a questionaire asking if we would attend depending on a bunch of considerations. Must all attendees get vaccinated before coming and show proof of it? Should all attendees get immediate covid tests at the front gate? Should everyone be required to wear masks at all times? The crowds can sometimes get pretty big, so how will there be social distancing, if at all. All of this is up in the air and I'm waiting for the final decision by the organizers of Burning Man before I make my decision. In November the Gerontological Society of America, of which I am a member and which focuses on research in gerontology, is supposed to meet in Phoenix. Last year it was cancelled, but if it happens this year it's unclear if they will have the same requirements as the possible Burner requirements given above. For all of these, the problem is the same. I can't take off from work without planning. I'll need someone to cover my practice (4-5 days for conventions,

2 weeks for Burning Man), and fronting the money for registration, hotels, transportation, etc. These aren't the biggest problems I'll have to worry about this year, considering the epidemic is still raging, but these are steps in getting back to normal. We'll see. temp today 98.6

Journal of the Plague Years, Day 308. I usually write about my own experiences, but I came across something in the scientific literature that might be important later. The January 15 issue of Science magazine had an article about covid in the Brazilian city of Manaus in the Amazon. I couldn't follow all the statistics in the article, but I'll try a summary. Using antibody tests they found that the covid infection rate by about October 2020 was about 76%, well above the herd immunity level. But people were still getting covid. At first non-pharmacological interventions (NPIs) were not used much and infection of the population and death increased dramatically. But even when the high infection rates were achieved, they only started coming down with NPI being implemented (there were no vaccines at that time). In other words, allowing the infection to run rampant achieved the theoretical herd immunity level, but didn't stop continued infection. Only NPIs eventually helped. This is similar I think to what happened in Sweden but worse. Sweden showed you couldn't reach herd immunity before you had to switch to NPIs. Manaus showed that even if you did reach herd immunity levels it might not have snuffed out the virus spread completely. This is the first report I've seen in the general scientific literature although there might be more detailed reports someplace else. If it comes out in the Times, remember you heard it here first. Does this mean it's hopeless? No, tune in tomorrow. temp today 98.3

Journals of the Plague Years, Day 309. The Great Race. There are two major trends, one actual and one theoretical that will determine what is going to happen with covid. One trend will make things better, the other will make it worse. The improvement trend exists because the number of cases of covid have decreased by almost 50% now that the Holiday spikes have receded. A smaller decrease in hospitalizations and deaths have occurred, but these can get steeper within the next 2-4 weeks, at least. Also, the number of people getting vaccinated is increasing, though slowly. Both of these are real and could significantly improve outcomes. The worsening trend consists of a few things. Mutant strains of covid are slowly entering the US and they might be more contagious and deadly, though we're not exactly sure how much. Some of the cable TV medical experts say there is a possibility of a fourth spike in cases by the summer if the worst projections about these mutants come true. We don't know how strong will immunity be in the long run, whether from vaccine or natural infection. If it fades fast, or if the mutants evade our immune systems, things could get worse. Some public health experts worry about a Super Bowl spike. To paraphrase a line from either the Bible or the play "A Man for All Seasons", it profit a man not to sell his soul for the whole world, but for Kansas City and Tampa! And, unfortunately, some states are actually banning mandatory face mask and distancing regulations. It's unclear if any of these possible problems will make the trends go down, but that is the choice. Hope that present good news and improvement continues and hope that future downward trends don't happen. We'll see. temp today 98.9

Journal of the Plague Years, Day 312, Monday Feb 8. I try to write these posts from my own personal experience, from the trenches in NYC. But sometimes things happen that I have to comment on before they hit NYC. Public health people had been warning that there should not be relaxation of covid precautions during Super Bowl Parties. Today, all over the news there are pictures of people in Tampa partying without masks or any other precautions. I hope they will be around to celebrate after next year's Super Bowl, but probably some won't. Florida has consistently violated precautions. A recent video of a market in Naples Florida showed almost no masks among customers or workers. Florida's vaccination program has received extensive criticism for sloppy guidelines and execution. Half of the

English mutant covid cases in the country are in Florida. People in the US travel and the cases in Florida don't stay in Florida. Later in the week some posts on people who are actually doing the right things. But in Florida, not so much. temp today 97.9

Journal of the Plague Years, Day 313. I've been relatively lucky during this plague. At the start I lost one friend and two patients. Recently, another patient who was in rehab. But several of my close relatives who were infected have all survived, so it hasn't hit me as hard as many others. The other day, coming into my building I asked the doorman how it was going and he said "just another day". The panic of March and April has been replace with the day to day routine of February. People are still running around hunting for vaccines, getting sick, dying, but so much of life is now becoming routine and even boring. The attractions of the city: dining, dining with friends, parties, subversive meetings, opera, theater, ballet, museums, and, for some, crowded athletic events have been put on hold to return at some time in the future. To be honest, boredom is preferable to panic and dreed. Putting up with this, with micro improvements from day to day, will continue for a while. At least it will unless another spike (Super Bowl, Mutant strains, whatever) sets us back. We'll see. temp today. 98.3

Journal of the Plague Years, Day 314. I've been saying that I expect the city to bounce back after covid with businesses and residents taking advantage of lower rents. But I forgot about condos and co-ops. I just learned one of my co-op neighbors has moved to Florida. So, are they fleeing the city? My doorman, an excellent source of information, said that move outs this year were no greater than previous years. I guess selling a co-op/condo is a lot more work and a bigger decision than leaving a rental (unless the rental is rent controlled/stabilized). But when they do leave they might be losing money. One of the throw away free community papers is called Our Town and has a lot of articles of local interest. It also has a list apartment sales which includes downtown location, size of apartment, price, days it took to sell it, and if it got above or below asking price. Before covid, some places got below asking price and some above. Since covid, including today, almost every single apartment was selling below asking price, sometimes for almost 25% below. I don't know the city statistics, but this might show that co-op/condo prices are dropping just like rentals. So what happens when this is over? Buying an apartment is as big a deal as selling one so if there is a flood of people moving back into NYC, especially Manhattan, a bargain might be irresistable. When I bought my co-op 28 years ago I did it during a real estate dip, and it made the difference between affording it and having to wait. This might happen with people coming into NYC, both returnees and newbies, who are looking for bargains and a chance to live in Emerald City. We'll see. 98.3

Journal of the Plague Years, Day 315. Yesterday I got my second Pfizer vaccine. My ALF has 3 days for vaccine, 3 weeks ago, yesterday and three weeks from now. By the end of the day yesterday 90 or our 95 residents got vaccinated. Three weeks ago 36 out of 99 staff got vaccines, and yesterday those 36 and another 20 new people took the vaccine. But this only comes to 56 of 99. The media has reported that there is a lot of skepticism in minority communities about the vaccine and as many as 40% said they wouldn't take it. Our staff is about 90% minority so our experience is about the same as estimated by the media. There is plenty of inequality in healthcare but when treatments are made available skepticism won't protect you from the virus. Maybe the numbers will slowly get better with time. We'll see. temp today 98.5

Journal of the Plague Years, Day 316. Two days ago I got the second Pfizer vaccination and I only had a sore arm as a side effect. Or so I thought. Last night I had a 4 hour Zoom call that disrupted my normal night routine, including sleep, and only got a few hours in. This morning I was awoken by a phone call from my office asking how I was. I didn't know why they were worried about me and why they were calling on a Saturday.

It eventually dawned on me that it was Friday, not Saturday and I had slept through my alarm clock and internal alarm which often wakes me at 7 on my days off. I rushed into the office and started to catch up on my work, explained myself to the staff, and started to ask if anyone had side effects from the vaccine two days ago. About 10 people had one or more of the following: sore arm, sore joints all over, fatigue, extreme fatigue, chills, shaking chills, low temp, or just a wiped out feeling, but no breathing problems or anaphylaxis reactions. I'm not sure how many of the patients had the same, but I know there were a few. How much of this was the vaccine, the irregular evening the night before, or whatever, is hard to know. I can't remember ever oversleeping like this before. The good news is that everyone seemed ok by today. We'll see. If I wake up tomorrow thinking it's Friday then maybe the side effects are a little longer lasting than I thought. And, if there are any anti-v****** reading this, it is NOT a reason to avoid the vaccine. temp today 97.6

Journal of the Plague Year, Day 320, Tuesday Feb 16. Mardi Gras! I told you about people in Tampa partying after the Super Bowl, but one of our biggest celebration is Mardi Gras. What's happening there? Last year Mardi Gras went on as usual and that resulted in Louisiana having one of the worst covid outbreaks in the country. They learned their lesson. If you go to Youtube right now and look for Mardi Gras Live Stream you will see the French Quarter empty, where it would normally be packed. A live stream in NYC shows Times Square with more people that New Orleans. The state, or city, closed bars, streets, cancelled the numerous massive parades and basically emptied the city. So Tampa was reckless, and New Orleans, at least this year, was careful. In a month or so we will see, if data is available, which of these approaches gave good results and which produced a disaster. Let's hope for the best. temp today 97.9

Journal of the Plague Year, Day 321. I've posted about the potential recovery of NYC but we're not the only city that's doing this. New

Orleans is getting creative also in its resurrection. Yesterday I described how Mardi Gras was shut down. But supposedly a local resident, Megan Boudreaux decided to decorate her front yard with Mardi Gras type colors and displays. She put it on social media and it took off. A new virtual/internet Krewe was set up: The Krewe of House Floats (Krewes are the fraternal organizations that run the major parades). The decorations are colorful, on Mardi Gras and other themes, and a lot of videos are on Youtube. There are as many at 3,000 of these yard displays now. Some people have started to refer to this as "Yardi Gras". Some local marching bands, called Second Line Bands, are giving small performances on local blocks. Will this continue next year? One front yard had a sign that said "Reserved for 2022". This might even develop into an annual tradition with yard displays getting more elaborate and competitive each year, like the home owners in Dyker Heights Brooklyn who put up massive Christmas lights each year. It would be a nice tradition and silver lining in the middle of this bleak covid dark cloud. temp today 98.8

Journal of the Plague Year, Day 322. A less cheerful post today. There have been many reports of horrendous crimes in the subways including stabbings and murder. One guy killed two and wounded two just in one day. This Tuesday when coming from work at 5, there were 6 cops in the subway station at 110th and Central Park North. I can't remember when I saw these many in one place on the subway. Today there were two cops at 5 on the station at 96th and Broadway. With a dramatic drop in riders, there should have been a dramatic drop in crime, but there wasn't. I don't remember if the overall numbers or the numbers in proportion to riders is up, but there is still too much even by subway crime standards. 500 more cops have been assigned, possibly with more to come. Liberals like me blame coved related emotional and economic stress, half empty train stations, and the overall lack of mental health services considering so many of these attacks are by people with serious mental health problems. Lack of mental health services have been steadily worsening since the 1970s and this crises may have just been latest and worst one among many. Conservatives blame bail reform, release from jail for covid reasons, and defund the police movement. When covid has passed we will see if there is a drop, although it might not answer the question as there will still be poor mental health services for liberals to blame, and there will still be bail reform for conservatives to blame. I can't predict if crime will decrease in the subways or anywhere else when this is over. We'll have to just wait and see and try to figure it out in the future. Sorry, but no great insights here. temp today 97.7

Journal of the Plague Year, Day 323. The restaurants have started opening up again. First at 25% capacity and next week at 35%, although it's unclear why we're waiting a week. But, at least it's something. Over the last week I've eaten, indoors at several of my usual places. I have dinner early, so what I saw might not be representative of later eating. Of the four places I visited at 5-6 on Friday and Sunday, one was pretty empty (but I know it filled later), two were half empty and one was packed. Walking around the neighborhoods, the usual downtown streets, I also saw some half-empty and some packed. A few of the crowded ones looked to be well above the 25% and I'm not sure how they did this legally, or maybe not so legally. Hope they don't lose their liquor licenses. Some people on TV being interviewed said they were hesitant about indoor eating so maybe that's keeping a few places empty. Some restaurant owners said they want the 35% increased asap, so maybe there are still hungry dinners out there waiting to come in from the cold. Let's hope this trend continues before more places close for good. 35% can't be sustained forever. temp today 98.2

Journal of the Plague Years, Day 326, Monday Feb 22. I've tried to write about NYC resiliance using my random observations around the city. Yesterday I had a few more. At about 5 PM I walked along the river to Canal street and then across Canal to Orchard street for dinner. At the start of the pandemic the streets were so empty that I could cross the West

Side Highway (aka West Street) against the light without any risk from traffic. It was really empty. No more. Yesterday traffic on West street was just about normal heavy. On Canal street traffic going into the Holland tunnel was backed up for about 2 blocks, closer to normal I think. The license plates were about half and half New York and New Jersey. I don't know what the Jersey people were doing in Manhattan. Brunch, bars, restaurants, shopping, visiting relatives, weekend get away? Also, why were all these NYC cars going into Jersey at 5 on a Sunday? Any ideas fellow Facers? temp today 98.3

Journal of the Plague Years, Day 327. My trip along Canal street a few days ago reminded me of something else that had been in plan sight but I overlooked. Lots of small businesses are trying to survive in NYC but the smallest of the small are the sidewalk vendors along Canal and other streets. From about West Broadway to Broadway on the South side of Canal there are countless sidewalk vendors side by side selling pocket books, hats, watches, various accessories and paraphernalia. Presumably these are virtually all counterfeit. Most vendors are men, from their speech they sound African, and their items are laid out on blankets on the sidewalk. The blankets allow them to bundle up their wares quickly when police come by for anti-counterfeit raids. Customers stroll by, negotiate and purchase this stuff just about every weekend, including this last weekend in 30 degree weather. I'm not sure if this street market on Canal is as extensive as it was before covid, or if it's slowly recovering, but at least these few blocks seem to be recovering or maintaining their activities no matter what. More NYC resilience. temp today 97.6

Journal of the Plague Years, Day 328. Continuing my trip along Canal street, the next group after the Africans selling purses, there were a block or two of small Asian, presumably Chinese, women. They were along the stretch close to Chinatown. The had single page laminated sheets of pictures of watches and would show the pictures to people walking by. This way the watches could be hidden away in a nearby stash safe from police or any passing by fast running street thief who decided to take advantage of these petite women. When a deal was made between a customer and seller someone would run to the stash, get the item, and make the individual sale without having to have all the items themselves on display. As with the other vendors, I don't know if these women were more numerous than before covid, but I know they were in the same location, and a whole bunch of them. temp today 98.0

Journal of the Plague Years, Day 329. (A little late). My final report on Canal street, for now. At the Eastern end on Canal near Mott and Elizabeth streets the collection of street vendors changed to produce stands. Lots of veggies and fruits and many stands selling them. All the vendors appeared to be Chinese. The two or three blocks on this stretch looked pretty crowded, especially considering the 30 degree weather, but I couldn't tell how this compared to the pre covid level of activity. Coming back from Orchard street after dinner, about 6 PM on Sunday evening, there were very few produce stands on Grand street. I'm pretty sure this was a lot less than previous Sunday nights but it was freezing out. So, one part of Canal either maintaining or resuming street vending and one part of Grand missing most of it. As the weather warms up I'll have a better idea if things are back to normal. Between people selling counterfeit luggage, fake watches and fresh produce another example of New Yorkers trying to hold on until this is all over. temp today 98.1

Journal of the Plague Years, Day 330. Enough of Canal street, now back up to the ALF where I work. Nationally, most assisted living facilities have about an 80% occupancy rate, 20% empty rooms. Where I work, Vista on 5th usually had 100% occupancy and a waiting list of a few months. Maybe because we accept Medicaid, which most places don't, maybe because of our location across from Central Park on 5th Avenue, or maybe because of a right level of services including a primary care geriatrician (yours truly) on site. That was before covid. Our loss of patients due to death or transfer to a nursing home has been 2-3 per month for the last year, which is about normal. But, nobody has been coming in. They might be thinking that ALFs have the same dire outcomes as nursing homes, and going into one was a death sentence. So, our occupancy rate dropped to 80% for the first time since opening in 2000. This week it may have turned around with three admissions this week and two next week. What's more, most were enthusiastic about moving in. Instead of "I don't want to be here but my children insisted I move in" we got "I'm so happy to be here, so there are people who could help me if I need it." Isolation and problems caused by covid drove people to desperation and resulted in a much more positive view of alfs. Let's hope this continues and we fill up completely. We have a good program and there are plenty of people who will benefit from it. temp today 98.3

Journal of the Plague Years, Day 333, Monday March 1. I recently wrote about seeing a bunch of police in the subway station near my job, 110th street and Central Park North. Since then I've see cops at train stations about a half dozen times, usually in groups of 3 or 4 or more. Sometimes this is early in the AM, which is very unusual, and sometimes during the evening rush hour. There has been a rise of some crimes in the subways for a while, but the recent attack on 4 people, with 2 deaths, finally got the city to move more cops into the subway. I don't know if this will help if the basic mental health services aren't improved also since a disproportionate numbers of these attacks seem to be by people with mental health problems of some type or another. Maybe some outreach into the subways before attacks by mental health or social workers might help instead of just cops. Is it covid, half empty train stations, general crime increases or general mental health deterioration that is causing this? We might not know until covid quiets down, whenever that will be. temp today. 98.8

Journal of the Plague Years, Day 334. In my ALF the residents have been off and on quarantine since covid started, and some are getting very stressed. Those with anxiety are more anxious, those with depression more depressed and those with dementia more demented and sometimes out of control. Today we got a new mental health group call Tapestry which will be counseling remotely to help us with psych med management. They will also help strengthen the two psychologists who are now coming in to do one on one counseling with some of our residents. We can use all the help we can get with mental health services. And we are in a secure enclosed environment. It's not surprising that people with mental health problems out on the streets, in the shelters, in the subways, etc, who get inadequate mental health services are having even more bizarre and sometimes deadly outbursts. I hope this gets better, even if only a little better, when covid is over. temp today 98.3

Journal of the Plague Years, Day 335. Yesterday I posted about the residents of my alf who were doing poorly. But, there are others. I just noticed that there is a sub-population of residents who are doing well in spite of quarantine and isolation: artists. We have at least 3 or 4 people who were professional artists before retirement and they still manage to do a lot of artwork. They all have studio apartments yet they have all managed to set up small easels and work spaces where they can still paint or draw. They stay in their rooms, seldom complain, and spend large amounts of time creating new art. They seem perfectly happy with being left alone to create their artwork. There are also a few amateur painters who are doing the same. By amateur I don't mean poor art, which I'm not qualified to judge, but they didn't work as artists before retirement. Retirement has now given them the time and opportunity to explore an interest they never had time for earlier. This calming effect of engulfing themselves in art, professional or amateur, might be one of the reasons that most alfs and nursing homes have art therapy. Sometimes this can be more effective for mental health than professional psychotherapy or the pills I give them. I hope that the museums can open soon so our residents, and I, can enjoy them again. Look at some of the drawings in my Facebook site by Avi Farin and you'll have an idea of the quality of the art being done. Long live art. temp today. 98.8i

Journal of the Plague Year, Day 336. Trying to restore normalcy is an ongoing theme of these posts. Here's more. At my alf we will soon have an exercise physiologist, a position about which I knew nothing. But our Rehab director Alexia said that he will be able to run small exercise classes of about 6 safely spaced people at a time either in the library or in the hallways of each individual floor. He can also act as a personal trainer for some of the people who have exhausted physical therapy Medicare services. I've posted about mental deterioration during quarantine, but there is also physical deterioration. Normally people are in and out of their rooms walking around to get meds, go to meals, attend events, or taking walks outside the building. Now they just sit around their apartments for extended periods getting weaker and weaker. These exercise classes should try and address a little of this. this is a new service we hope can expand as the quarantine slowly, very slowly, loosens. Every little bit helps, if only 6 people at a time. temp today 97.1

Journal of the Plague Years, Day 337. Is recently posted that when vaccines were given at my alf, about 95% or residents and 60% of staff took the vaccine. I was disappointed that only 60% of the staff took it. I know that there is distrust of the vaccine in minority communities and out staff is about 90% minority. But these vaccines were at work so people would not have to find a location to get the shots, and they were free. So, I thought there would be a higher %. I've just found out that nursing homes might have had even worse numbers. A recent report by the DOH (Department of Health, not D'OH of Homer Simpson), said that nursing home staff has only had a 37% vaccine. I don't know if they are comparable, since I don't know if the 60% vs 37% takes into account who got both shots and who got one shot, but it still looks that my place might not be so bad after all. If the staff responded a little better than average for other long term care workers, then maybe they will continue to respond and get up to the 95% vaccination rate of our residents. We'll see. temp today 98.2

Journal of the Plague Years, Day 340, Monday March 8. How often do you see a Starbucks closed? On Bleeker street one closed before covid but it had the misfortune of being two storefronts away from Rocco's Pastry so it may have been doomed anyway. But the one on Hudson and Tenth street looked healthy. It was one of the first places to open when take out orders were allowed. There were usually a few people in front, at least in the mornings, who had ordered from their phone apps and picked up their orders later. Looked good for a while. This week they closed. Maybe because there are a few other Starbucks within walking distance. Maybe because their prime corner location also came with a prime rent and their landlord wasn't about to give a cash cow like Starbucks get a brake. Or maybe because of the competition on the same block. More tomorrow. 98.1

Journal of the Plague Years, Day 341. Starbucks on this block just died but there are two possible accomplices who did this. On the other end of the same block is Blackstone Coffee Roasters which provides upscale coffee and nosh for what looks like an upscale clientele of young people, at least in the mornings and lunchtime. In the middle of the block is Hudson Deli and Grocery, which I've described before. It is a family run place opened 24/7 run by Egyptian Copts. When I go there on the weekends for morning coffee and bacon/egg/cheese sandwich there are usually maybe one or two people there. Constant turnover, but never a long line. I asked the counter person if Starbucks closing helped them and she said it didn't make a difference. That's because their main business is during the week when school kids and their parents going to PS 3 one block away stop in for coffee and breakfast, lunch, and after school snacks. That business is keeping them open, and it was completely invisible to me because I was never around those times. So, what did I learn from this? One, there may be major things happening, even on the grass roots level, that make the difference between survival and closing. This might be happening all over, so if other Facers see unobserved trends happening, in NYC or wherever, don't hesitate in posting. Second, there are symbiotic relationships that are really significant. A deli surviving and a school opening, even partially, support each other financially and nutritionally and emotionally in a city that's still struggling. These visible but subtle connections must be countless in a city this size and complexity. I'll keep looking for more. temp today 98.7

Journal of the Plague Years, Day 342. Let's keep on the food theme for now, it's a lot lighter than talking about illness and death. Within walking distance of my house there are four places I often patronized that have closed. Bethel Gourmet deli was a small traditional deli across from St. Vincent's/Aids Memorial park and I would sometimes grab a coffee and pastry after work and sit in the park. Sweet Corner on Hudson and Charles would be for Sat or Sun morning with a coffee and blueberry muffin. Philip Marie was a nice restaurant where I sometimes went for brunch on the weekends. Westville on tenth street was a branch of a chain of Westvilles that had good inexpensive food, and they delivered. I don't know if the other branches in Chelsea or Hudson Square deliver. Four places, all food oriented, are a small loss considering everything else happening with this pandemic, and if these are the only losses it would be great. Facers reading this: post any of your favorites that are gone before we forget them. temp today

Journal of the Plague Years, Day 343. Yesterday I spoke about what closed, today what's opened. During the height of the pandemic new places have opened in the neighborhood also. In the space left over by Two Boots which has relocated from 7th avenue and Greenwich avenues to Sheridan square is a new pizza place called Zazzy's. It is an offshoot of one on Orchard street and makes both traditional and vegan pizza. But the main new addition is Dante's West, on Hudson and Perry. It is an offshoot of Dante's cafe which was an old time Italian cafe before it became a very hip, expensive, and crowded martini bar. The new branch, a few blocks from my home, has a similar vibe and is often packed. When the weather is tolerable the outside tables are filled from brunch to dinner, and the inside tables usually crowded at all times. I may have mentioned this place a while back when it closed on Saturday nights because the crowds were too big and they didn't want to lose their liquor license like the White Horse Tavern. Now they're open and probably doing more business than the four places I mentioned yesterday that closed combined. These are all food places. There are also lots of small shops, especially cute expensive clothing stores on Bleeker including Whalebone on Christopher. I don't know all these stores, but I think there are a lot of them and many have opened during the pandemic. I thought that when all this was over the city would rebound. But, some of the rebounding might have already started. Any more uplifting stories like this would be most welcome, from inside the city or wherever. temp today 98.7

Journal of the Plague Years, Day 344. I wanted to end the week on an up note and describe some of the good news at the ALF where I work. But I found something even more uplifting, although more subjective. As I was walking from my office on Fifth Avenue and 108th street to the subway on 110th and Lenox, I passed Central Park. It was loaded with people. The somewhat warmer weather, even with a mild chilly breeze, had attracted mobs of people. Kids, parents, bike riders crowded all the open areas in that little corner of Central Park. There was an ice cream truck, the first of the season I think, on 110th street with a line of kids and mothers waiting for ice cream. The whole scene was so idyllic I almost forget we were still in a pandemic. The small number of people wearing masks and the cops at the entrance to the subway brought me back to reality, but even that couldn't dampen the joy, yes joy, at seeing so many people out and about. If I knew how to do the video on my phone and post it, I would have a much better image to share with you all, and it would go way beyond my mere words. This can't be the only place this is happening. Those of you who are more video competent than I am, which is probably all of you, are invited to video, or at least photo, similar scenes in the parks, beaches, and open spaces that are coming out of hibernation. If you capture an ice cream truck, that counts for extra points. temp today. 98.7

Journal of the Plague Years, Day 347, Monday March 15. I don't know if this pandemic has made me hyper vigilant but today's post is about garbage. I've noticed recently that sidewalk trash baskets appear overfilled more often. I don't remember what it was like before covid, but I do notice a lot of filled baskets now. I read that when NYC's budget started to tank, there was a cut in Sanitation department's budget for sidewalk trash basket collections by over 50% (I read this in The Post, so take it with a grain of salt) Last weekend I saw something I've never seen before. On the corner of Bleeker and Christopher two corners had single baskets and two corners had double baskets, everyone of the 6 completely filled. I've never ever seen double baskets on corners in all my years in NYC. Was this just an oversight? Was this done intentionally so that garbage collectors could pick up more at every corner? Like a Qanon conspiracy nut, or an internet troll trying to find some hidden connection in random websites, I might be over interpreting this observation. I called 311 to ask if anyone at the Department of Environmental Protection, the DEP, knew about this and nobody was aware of it. This was only one corner of many. But, if you see this yourself, or read about it anywhere, remember you heard it here first. temp today 98.3

Journal of the Plague Years, Day 348. Lots of my observations have been about food places. Walking around Sunday I realized that there are other types of stores in NYC. Who knew? I walked across Houston street on Sunday evening about 4 PM and saw a line in front of a clothing store called Vintage. Further down the street in front of REI camping equipment there was another long line. And I know from other trips that the Supreme store on the Bowery often has lines down the block. I thought they just sole skateboards and back packs, but they also have a lot of clothing items. Since my mom worked in a garment sweatshop almost all of her life, you would think I would be more aware of the garment industry. Apologies to clothing mavens and fashionistas everywhere for overlooking this essential part of NYC industry which suffered as much from covid as anywhere else. Good luck to them all, and Facers reading this should feel free to give some input on these types of stores above and beyond my tiny contribution. temp today 97.9

Journal of the Plague Years, Day 349. Today, St. Patrick's Day, was my first happy hour in about a year. The place was Lucky, a bar on avenue B between 10th and 11th. This is also my first Burning Man happy hour in a year. Burners sometimes have an anarchist tendency and so I was worried about the rules covering bars would be ignored, but I was wrong. Abby, the owner, was meticulous in enforcing them, at least until 7 when I left. The bar itself, inside, was completely closed, no seats or tables. The back yard had tables as did the sidewalk/curbside outside. There was still adequate space between people, and people were actually wearing masks when not eating or drinking. Speaking of eating and drinking, I had a traditional two glasses of Guinness (which I usually drink) and corned beef and cabbage meal (which I seldom eat, except on St. Patrick's day). It wasn't completely normal as she had asked for reservations or no people sitting one at a table, we had to be in groups. I introduced myself to Mike, a local resident, world traveler and published poet (yes, they do get published now and then) and we shared a table and a few drinks. Lucky is a friendly place and it was common to meet old friends and new ones before this all started. So, I hope it's not a year for my next happy hour. There are lots of friends to see again or meet, lots of Guinness to drink, but maybe not so much corned beef and cabbage until next year. temp today 98.5

Journal of the Plague Years, Day 350. I've been posting about small businesses either closing or opening. What about large businesses? I'll need help with local posters on this but it involves a big closed store on 7th avenue. On 7th avenue between 12th and 13th street on the east side of the street there is a massive closed store. It used to have a chain drug store that almost took up the whole block. But, I'm not sure if it closed during the pandemic or if it closed before. On Google maps its name wasn't listed on the map so it might have been closed for a while, maybe before this all started. It was a very big place and must have paid a fortune in rent, so it wouldn't be surprising if it closed a while ago and I just didn't notice. It also might have closed at the start of the lockdown. Anyone who knows, please let me know. Other chain stores, like the Rite Aid on Hudson and Charles, are still open so somehow their deep pockets are getting them through the bad times. I've tried to do these posts based on my observations, but there might be things I've missed right in front of me, like a big drug store in front of the subway a pass through twice a day. Let me know. temp today 97.8

Journal of the Plague Years, Day 351. I'm ending the week on a good note, as I try to do, and will describe some mostly good news from my ALF. We operate under DOH rules and the last week or so they gave us a break. Visitors to the facility were allowed in to see family members, meetings of up to 10 people are ok (for exercise classes, yoga, discussion groups and of course, bingo), as is sitting in the lobby, spaced, but out of their solitary confinement and with others. This is a significant improvement over the isolation of just a few weeks ago. But, a problem soon appeared. One of our staff members tested positive, the second one in a month. We knew that with 40% of staff not taking the vaccine this would happen. So, we had to go on partial lock down with outside visitors banned but many of the other internal activities allowed as long as there was no mixing with outsiders. Fortunately, there was a loophole in this rule with "compassionate visits" for those residents who were really sick. The exact guidelines are unclear to me, other than to note that things are complicated, with old strict rules, new relaxation of the rules, re-establishment of rules when somebody tests positive and then loopholes in those re-established rules. What a mess! But the overall tendency seems to be slowly opening up again with two steps forward and one step back, or something like that. We're looking forward to three steps forward and no steps back. Soon, I hope. temp today 98.9

Journal of the Plague Year, Day 354, Monday March 22. A few weeks ago I posted about the South side of Canal street and the numerous sidewalk vendors. Yesterday I went to the North side of Canal. There were lots of sidewalk vendors, those with their wares spread out on the sidewalk and those with laminated cards showing their goods. There were also lots of store fronts. From Sixth avenue to Chrystie street I counted 108 store fronts. About half were closed and I couldn't tell which were permanently closed and which just closed for Sunday. The opened stores included a half dozen banks, a few sit down restaurants but plenty of fast food and convenience delis, and many souvenir and jewelry places selling knockoff trinkets, t-shirts, perfumes, watches, etc. I don't know if this array was better or worse than before coved. But I do know that the sidewalk was filled with people. If I didn't know about the epidemic I would be hard pressed to tell the difference between this and any other Sunday afternoon. That's the good news. The bad news is that many people along Canal, and the Hudson River park I walked through going down there, weren't wearing masks. The sunny weather, breeze, and fresh air made outdoor walking seem safe. I hope we're not getting too over confident or we'll be paying for it with our lives. OK, that's a little morbid, so let's just hope the maskless people are right and this pessimist is wrong. temp today 98.3

Journal of the Plague Years. Here is another unusual, maybe trivial, observation that may or may not be significant. Last week when I was taking a taxi coming home, the driver asked me if I wanted to ride off the meter. I can't remember the last time I was in a yellow cab that kept the meter off. It was years, maybe decades, ago and to hear the driver suggest it shocked me. I agreed, gave him his requested fee and a tip also. Is this significant? It was only one driver on one trip. Is it a response to covid or the overall poor state of the yellow cab drivers? If anyone else in NYC has or had a similar experience let me know. One case is anecdotal, two is a coincidence, and three is a trend. If you more people have a similar experience then we have discovered a new trend which may or may not be a response to covid. temp today 98.2

Journal of the Plague Years, Day 256 (I forgot to label yesterday as 255). The taxi story from yesterday is maybe a way someone is trying to survive covid financially, however he was doing it. There are other recent examples. The shoe shine place in Penn Station cut their hours from 9 a day to 5, staff from 6 to two and prices up from $5 to $8. Astor haircutters, after being saved from closure by a local investor, raised their haircut price on Sunday afternoons from $20 to $25. These aren't massive increases for someone with a good steady income, like me. And stretching out shoe shines or haircuts are is always possible. But I wonder about similar increases in necessary items, like food, healthcare and rent (when eviction bans expire) for people with much more limited income. If you notice any increases, please post them so we can all see if these increases are big, small, or non-existent. temp today 98.2

Journal of the Plague Years, Day 257. There is a lot of anecdotal talk about people leaving NYC to avoid the plague. One of the places they, including our beloved former President, flee to is Florida. This isn't just a spontaneous movement but there are incentives. I recently got a cold mailing from some medical group in Florida trying to recruit MDs to come to Florida. Specifically, they wanted me to relocate to The Villages which is probably the largest senior community in the US. They describe a good deal medically, although they don't mention salary, but it sounds like I would have plenty of time to see patients, plenty of support services, and the joy of living in the middle of Florida. Besides the fact that this is a heavily R********* district, and I would probably get into a political argument every single day I'm there, another reason exists. I grew up in the Bronx, always feeling bad that I would never afford to live in Manhattan, or "The

City" as we called it. Now, my own work and fate has put me in Greenwich Village, and I'm not likely to change anytime soon. But leaving NYC to go to a maskless, clueless, spring break superspreader state is pretty inconceivable. I feel sorry for the suckers who decided to move and went from the frying pan into the fire, just as Fla tempts fate with another potential spike in cases. If I had more time to go into details about my move from the Bronx to Manhattan I would, but let me just say, in the words of an old TV show, "There are 8 million stories in the Naked City, and this has been one of them." temp today 98.3

Journal of the Plague Year, Day 258. I try to end the week on a positive note, and I'm not sure if today's is positive or still unclear. Before covid the ALF where I worked would be inspected by the state every year or two. They went over the dining room, medication room, medical records, fire safety and just about everything. Every 2-3 years there would be an inspection by the health inspectors (not sure if they were from the state or city), and they would mostly inspect the dining room. Since covid, that has changed. The state hasn't been back, but skipping a year isn't too unusual. But the health inspectors have been around every three months, which is unprecedented. They look at the dining room, make sure everyone is wearing the proper protective equipment throughout the building, even making sure the hallways have stickers on the floor every 6 feet to show people how to space themselves. This looks pretty intimidating, but the inspectors are not unreasonable, as some used to be. They know everyone is having a hard time coping and they are flexible, but clear, about the enforcement of rules. This keeps us very much on our toes. We don't know when it will end, but we do very well on the inspections and haven't gotten into any significant trouble. That's good news, but when this all ends it will be even better. temp today 98.5

Journal of the Plague Years, Day 261, Monday March 29th. The more walks I take around the city the more details I see that I had missed. I've spoken about lines at various types of stores, and here's another one. Dessert places sometimes have really long lines. Not the sit down pastry shops, but grab and go places. When walking along Bleeker last night I saw a few ice cream or pastry shops with a few people outside. On Orchard street there is a place that makes ice cream from oat milk, whatever that is, and there were over 20 people in line. Coming back, there were about a dozen people lined up at Eileen's cheesecake on Cleveland Place. So they were line up for new trendy gourmet sweets along with old school cheesecake. Is this because covid has made us frantic for guilty sweet pleasures, or has this been going on all along? When all of this is over, I'll try and take another look at some of these and other places and see what was baseline NYC food frenzy and was was a covid induced need for caloric hedonism. temp today 97.6

Journal of the Plague Year, Day 262. Those of you who have been reading these posts know that I enjoy scooping the NY Times on some covid issue. A few weeks ago I posted how my facility had provided vaccines to residents and staff. 95% of residents took it but only 60% of staff. Yesterday in The Times they had an article "One Nursing Home Mission, To Convince Its Hesitant Staff." There had been word of mouth around the ALF community that other places had similar results, but this article confirmed it. It also outlined incentives, like encouragement, staff training, or gifts, to increase staff vaccinations. I'm not sure how fast staff vaccines are increasing, if at all, at any facility including my own. When quarantine regulations are eliminated, at some time in the future, we may no longer be required to wear masks at work. If the state requires non-vaccinated staff to continue wearing masks, which is what they now do with flu shots, then possibly a lot more staff will get their shots. This is what happened with flu shots, so maybe it will happen with covid shots. We'll see, although I don't know how long it will take to reach this point, or if it will still be needed. temp today 97.5

Journal of the Plague Years, Day 263. Since this series of posts started on April 1 last year, today should be day 265, not 263. somewhere along the way I miscounted and lost a few days. Hold on while I go back and recheck the last years posts and find it......ok, only kidding. What's lost is lost. Let's readjust this post count so that today is day 265. I've added a few leap days to make it accurate. Tomorrow I'll start with day 266. I didn't think this would all take more than a year of posts, but here we are and things are still going on. So, this post is more of an anniversary than a content filled post, which will resume tomorrow. I hope I don't have to keep counting days for another year. This is beginning to go from interesting to gruesome. temp today. 98.6

Journal of the Plague Years, Day 266 (adjusted for the missing two days). The head of the CDC says she has a foreboding of impending doom when she looks at the recent covid numbers. For months the disease rate plummeted, then leveled off, and now starting to rise. She is looking at the national numbers, but I'm down in the trenches on a practical level and I'm starting to get the same feeling. For months we had no new cases at the ALF where I work. Then we had a cases isolated by weeks in between. This last week we had three new cases on the same day. Two were from unvaccinated staff members and one from a fully vaccinated resident who makes many trips out of the facility and probably caught it outside. All were put on isolation, all were asymptomatic. The CDC recently said vaccinated people can't transmit the virus but this patient had a positive test, which was done twice. I don't know if his positive test means he can transmit, or if it just colonizes him. But, it's frightening, and maybe even a foreboding of impending doom. It's only three weeks of so-so numbers and one week of bad numbers, so maybe it's not a disaster yet. Or, maybe it is. temp today 97.4

Journal of the Plague Years, Day 267. I try to end the week on an up note, but this week that's been hard. So, I'll go back to a previous positive post, although it's not entirely positive. About a week or two ago the state DOH said we could start having visitors at our ALF. But, there were a few rules we had to follow. This week I got a list of them. There are at least 12 rules of behavior. God only needed 10 commandments to tell us what to do, but I guess life is more complicated now and the DOH needs 12. They include making appointments ahead of time instead of just walking in, age limits, time limits, staff member to enforce social distancing rules, temp and illness check on entry, bathroom restrictions (!), and a few others. We, I guess it's better to have visitation with a dozen rules than no visits with only one rule: STAY OUT, which is what will happen if we keep getting new covid infections. temp today 97.3

Journal of the Plague Year, Day 370, Monday April 5. A lot of my posts have been about restaurants, large and small, and the negative impact of covid. There may be a positive impact also. Several of my favorite places have outdoor tables. Seating can be as much as 25-50% of indoor seating, even when indoor seating is allowed to go back to 100% of capacity. When covid is over, whenever that is, these places will have seating capacity of 125 to150% of pre-covid capacity. This will potentially enable them to make up income lost during the lockdown. Maybe. This depends on enough people coming out to eat instead of staying home with GrudHub or actually cooking. It also depends on whether the total number of seats is too large. If all these places open up but can only fill a fraction of their seats, they might start running into trouble after covid. In the best of times, restaurants are very competitive and there is constant turnover. Half empty places might make it worse. We won't know until covid is gone and the surviving places, along with newbies, try and keep going. Save your money and get ready to dine out. It will help keep NYC, although not our waistlines, in good shape. temp today 98.3

Journal of the Plague Years, Day 371. I read that the vaccine is now available to people 16 years old and older. It was just a news story, along with all the others, until I came home from work today at 5 PM. Outside of the Lenox Hill Village ER there was a long line around the corner and down the block. For those who don't know it, the Lenox Hill Village ER is a free standing full ER that is not physically connected to a hospital but is affiliated with Lenox Hill Hospital a few mile uptown. It is very modern and provides almost all the services a regular ER does. All the people on line were young, not a single gray haired individual that I could see. There was a story that the ER was charging ER rates of a thousand bucks for a simple vaccine shot but I haven't seen that confirmed yet and I don't know if that's the bill they send to the insurance company or what. I couldn't see any millenials or younger ones paying that for a vaccine. Whatever the cost, there they were. I'll see over the next few days if the crowds go down, but it was an impressive sight. temp today 97.6

Journal of the Plague Years, Day 372. A view from the subways. One of the new developments on the subways is the presence of lots of cops. In the last twenty or so subway trips (two a day, 4 days a week) about 4-5 days police were on the platform or just outside the entrance. This might not seem like a lot, but before that mentally ill person stabbed four, killing two, you almost never saw police in the subway. Most of the ones I've seen are at the 110th street and Central Park North station or 14th street, in both cases on the 2 and 3 lines. I don't know what effect this has had since attacks on the subway seem to be still occurring. Eventually some data will come out and we'll see if these attacks are more or less than before the police surge about a month ago. Meanwhile the rest of the subway seems the same. temp today 97.6

Journal of the Plague Years, Day 373. (A little late) More on subways. When I said the rest of the subway is getting back to normal, that's only half true. In a typical week there will be 2 or 3 beggars, homeless people sleeping and lying on the seats, and obviously mentally ill people. 2 or 3 of each category, not 2 or 3 all together. I think this is less then what was happening before they started closing at night and before the recent police surge, although it's hard to remember exactly. It wasn't the kind of thing I was paying attention to a year ago. One thing that hasn't gotten back to normal is Times Square. The station is still relatively empty and more people get off the train there then get on. So, the tourist crowd, theater crowd, and office workers have not returned, and nobody knows when and if they will. temp today 98.4

Journal of the Plague Years, Day 374. It's Friday and time to be upbeat again. Good news at my ALF. Our beautiful dining room which is on the top floor, 14 stories above Fifth Avenue, will reopen on Monday. It has been closed since last March. It is one of the nicest amenities of the facility with a view of Central Park while residents have their meals. There will be a little re-arranging to insure social distancing, but it will be enjoyed by everyone there, except for a few residents who have really gotten into hermit mode during the quarantine. Even better, the DOH guidelines have changed so that if an individual staff member or resident tests positive for covid, only that person will go on isolation and the whole facility will not have to shut down, as was previously the case. This is good news and something to look forward to for next week. temp today 98.2

Journal of the Plague Years, Day 377, Monday April 12. The Daily News editorial page on Saturday had an editorial entitled "Journal of the Plague Year." Since I read the News, maybe somebody there reads my posts. Or maybe both of us stole that dramatic line from Daniel Defoe who wrote "A Journal of the Plague Year" in about 1666. Boccaccio wrote Decameron about the Black Death. There are probably other diaries of this type from ancient times since the Greeks, Romans, and Byzantines had plenty of history changing plagues to write about. Maybe the highly literate Facers reading this post can give me a few quotes from those times. It got me to thinking (usually a good thing) about why I write these posts. Communicating with a small circle of friends and relatives is beneficial in a time when quarantine has made communication difficult. Maybe it's to vent. Maybe it's vanity thinking my insights are profound. Maybe it's just to witness. Maybe it's to structure my evenings with self imposed homework. Maybe it will help a student in 2121 going for a Ph.D. in Community Health find obscure documentation of history before the cure was found for all Covid viruses. But, even if I can't figure it out now, I'll keep writing and try and figure it out later. Or maybe that Ph.D. student will figure it out. temp today 98.6

Journal of the Plague Years, Day 378. I've posted a lot about developments at the ALF where I work, but not so much about my own medical practice. My practice there started as a full time primary care geriatrics practice taking care of the residents of the facility. The facility is community run and non-profit but the practice was started by St. Vincent's hospital as an "outside vendor" renting space there like in any office building. When St. Vincent's went under St. Luke's took over the practice and they eventually merged with Sinai. I was part of the Sinai system until March 2020 and separated via a very messy divorce. I joined a medical group, Lyons Medical Care, and things looked good. Instead of 6-7 patients a day, a very low number compared to other practices, I thought I could get visits up to 8-10 a day. Not only would this allow me to see my patients for all their emergencies and routine visits, but possibly have monthly visits for preventive care. Then covid hit. Because of isolation protocols everything takes longer with putting on protective equipment, seeing patients in their rooms instead of my office, and other factors. Now I see 4-5 patients a day. Everything that must get done gets done, but it all takes more time. My practice doesn't run in the red and I still get a good income. But, if I'm seeing my patients less frequently then they're seeing their doctor less frequently and who knows what problems are developing that I won't see until there is a crisis. Another reason to hope for the end of this pandemic, asap. 98.0

Journal of the Plague Years, Day 379. I mentioned last week that our dining room was reopening. Here are some details. When we closed down March 2020 it was done quickly. Within a day or two, every resident was put on quarantine in their rooms and the staff was given a whole bunch of rules to follow about safety precautions while scrambling to get the equipment to do it. Opening up is going much more slowly. Our dining room usually has two seatings of 65 people each with shared tables close to each other. Now we are allowed two seatings of 10 people each, or twenty a day. Each day there are a different 20 residents until all the hundred current residents get one day in the dining room instead of in their own apartments. Each person has their own individual table spaced at least 6 feet from the next table. there are no shared tables yet. On Monday about 12 of the 20 actually showed up and Tuesday about 14 people. Others preferred to stay in their rooms. What effect did this have on the residents? tune in tomorrow. temp today 98.3

Journal of the Plague Years, Day 380 (A little late). I've only spoken to a few residents who ate in the dining room. A few of them loved it, getting out of their rooms into the bright sunshine. Another thought it weird when he and only one other person was in the large dining room. I'll have to ask around and see other people's opinions. One very promising outcome was noticed by the staff. The people who did eat there cleaned their plates. Maybe because these were people with big appetites but also maybe because eating with others, even when spaced 6 feet apart, in a nice setting with warm food served quickly is more enjoyable than being alone in your room, eating out of a container with cooled off and somewhat soggy food. We've been worried about a few residents who have been losing weight or getting dehydrated because of eating alone. We're going to make an effort to get these problematic eaters up to the dining room more and keep a close eye on their eating behavior. Food is more than just calories. Quality of life issues sometimes determines good nutrition vs just barely managing. temp today 98.4

Journal of the Plague Year, Day 381. After a few posts on the opening of the dining room, here is the final tally. About 70-75 residents out of about 100, came up to the dining room. Some didn't due to covid fears, habitually not liking the food, or just getting spoiled by having room service and strengthening their hermit like tendencies. But, I think 75% is pretty good for the first week. This might get better as people start to get into the habit of coming to the dining room, especially if dinner can be added to the lunches we have now. There's always a chance that the relative novelty of the dining room will wear off, or that the 6 foot spacing will weird out some people, but give it time. I think expanding these hours, once sufficient staff are retrained in covid precautions, will be better for the patients nutrition, hydration, and socialization (which should decrease depression, anxiety, and isolation). We'll see. temp today 98.5

Journal of the Plague Years, Day 384, Monday April 19. During my Sunday walk from my home to Orchard Street for dinner, I passed through Washington Square Park. I've often used the bathroom there on the south side of the park, as it is a convenient halfway point. Yesterday, when the park was packed with people at 4:30 I noticed a long line in front of the women's bathroom. This wasn't unusual, but there was also a long line in front of the men's room which I don't remember seeing before. Maybe it occurred and I never noticed it in pre-covid times, or it was just a coincidence. Like so many of these random observations I've been making around the city, and posting here, I don't know what's significant and covid related and what isn't. If any of these observations seem interesting to the Facers reading these posts, let us know. If not, just ignore these ramblings and find some cute cat playing the piano posts. temp today 98.7

Journal of the Plague Years, Day 385. When posting about the reopening of the city, I've talked a lot about over all improvements in numbers of restaurants and customers. Now for something more personal. This weekend I got together for indoor dining with three vaccinated friends at a restaurant. I had outdoor dining with three at the start of the quarantine, but none since. After a year it was a nice return to normal. Also, I'm talking to friends about going to the opera soon, the Met hopefully. I haven't been to an opera, ballet, Broadway show, museum, or even a movie since this all started. Work, zoom, individual dining, and my computer have prevented me from becoming a total hermit but that's not what I moved to Manhattan for. Culture and entertainment are opening, and between masks, vaccines, and maybe herd immunity, we'll all be able to enjoy them again. Soon. I hope. temp today 98.1 (This was a very positive post, I should have saved it for the Friday uplift.)

Journal of the Plague Years, Day 386. Continuing on the theme of opening up one person at a time, that goes for health stuff too. Health care workers, including doctors, are always warned to make sure we take care of ourselves while taking care of others. Over the last year I've remembered that rule, but like so many others, didn't follow it. Being so preoccupied with day to day problems and disasters I procrastinated a lot. I'm very good at it. Now I have to make up for lost time. Today I saw my own ENT doc (nothing serious, just ear wax), and my dentist will be in a few months if I can't get them to push up my appointment. My primary care physician is next if I can only get them to answer the phone. I hate making appointments over the internet but prefer to talk to an actual office staff person. I'm old fashioned that way, boomer that I am. Yes, even doctors have trouble making appointments. But, it will happen eventually, hopefully all covered by my Medicare, and there will be another step back to normal. Soon. I hope. temp today 98.0

Journal of the Plague Years, Day 387. One more step for opening up. tonight I had dinner with 7 friends, a going away party for a co-worker at Carmine's on upper Broadway. At least 7/8 were vaccinated and we were able to enjoy dinner without worry about covid. Very early in these posts I was very worried about people congregating at restaurants, without masks, talking to each other and maybe spreading covid. I was very worried. Things have changed and now it's safer and safer to get together in groups. Many other groups in the restaurant, after having their temperatures taken, were sitting around in groups without masks and seemed to be acting normally and enjoying themselves. Small groups getting together, if careful, can open things up more. Another positive sign. Let's hope it continues. temp today 98.0

Journal of the Plague Years, Day 388. (A little late). My usual upbeat Friday post is a little mixed today, but since the last few days of posts have been "reopening" themed and optimistic this will balance things off a little. At the begging of the year there was a tremendous drop in covid cases. About 2 months ago this stopped and there have been minor ups and downs in cases recently. The case numbers should be dropping to zero, but they aren't. Maybe it's because of vaccine fears, but more likely new mutant strains coming in and slipping by vaccine prevention. But, there is some very good news. Actual deaths, from the various internet public health sources, show that in the last two weeks or so actual deaths have gone from about 1000 a day to about 700. In spite of mutants, vaccine phobias, and persistent avoidance of NPIs (non-pharmacological interventions like masks, isolation, etc) the death rate is dropping. If this continues covid could be downgraded to a seasonal virus like the flu. Still deadly, but not overwhelming. We'll see. temp today 97.8

Journal of the Plague Years, Day 391, Monday April 26. Besides posting about the virus itself, I've also talked a lot about NYC renewal. One of the aspects of this is whether office work, and office occupancy, will return now that we are all used to using Zoom. Not only will the previous status be in doubt, but there are a lot of office buildings being built.

On Spring and Varick, I think, there is a tremendous full block empty lot announcing a commercial building expected in 2024. There another smaller lot on Broome and the Bowery. Google is in the St. John's Center. More being built on Broadway in the 90s. Can these be filled? NY Magazine this week has several articles on office work. Some articles are projections and guesses about the future, many are reminiscences of office workers who worked with famous people. But, on page 60 there is a list of predictions over the last 50 years about how "the office" is dead and people want to work from home. These predictions were all wrong. I hope that reports of "the office" being dead were greatly exaggerated. Most people are social animals and congregating is sometimes more productive than hermit like behavior, and sometimes even more enjoyable. temp today 98.5

Journal of the Plague Years, Day 392. More about crowds, following up on yesterday. Offices aren't the only institutions with a great potential for reopening. I've posted a lot about restaurants being filled up as soon as they were allowed to. People have always been able to see movies on cable or Netflix, but they still went to movies. They could get opera, ballet, and classical music on Youtube, but they still went out and pain high prices to sit in crowded concert halls. Broadway plays were packed, off and on depending on how hot the season was. Even dining attracts crowd lovers. Home delivery is cheap and easy, at least in the city, but people pack into crowded restaurants at high prices to eat. All this was true before covid I don't see why it won't happen again after this is over, at least mostly. I'm looking forward to see if my predictions are correct. If not, Facers reading this can point out my errors when the time comes. temp today 97.7

Journal of the Plague Years, Day 393. Yesterday I spoke about crowds getting back together. There's one crowd that won't. Burning Man has just been cancelled for this year. It is always the week before Labor Day and last year that was the peak of the epidemic. This year the rate of disease should be much less. But, there was no way to know for sure. To build the infrastructure for 75,000 or so people, sell tickets, recheck the state (Nevada) and Fed regulations, etc. is a lot of work that has to be done many months ahead of opening day. Many of Burning Man's activities take place in the open air in the sunlight but there are also plenty of times when people are crowded together in tents or RVs, and when the Man burns at the end, there are tens or thousands of people together shoulder to shoulder for several hours. There is no way of knowing how many of those people will be vaccinated, how widespread the mutant strains will be, how many people who do get sick can be taken care of in the several medical tents there or how many will have to travel a few hours to Reno, and how many hospital beds will be available in Reno. Too much to plan four months in advance. And regardless of how anarchistic Burning Man might seem, the organizers are very careful about safety. So, all eyes on 2022 when everything will be safer. It will be safer, won't it?

Journal of the Plague Years, Day 394. I've posted about the race between vaccines vs viruses. Recently, good news and bad. Good news is that NYC is under 2% new cases and bars and restaurants will be opening a lot in the next few weeks. The bad is that Staten Island is the only part of NYC at about 3%. Why there? It is the most conservative part of NYC and I hope right wing types aren't taking this anti-v** cultural loyalty test too seriously. It might seem like poetic justice for anti-******* to get sicker than the general population but I being conservative shouldn't produce a death sentence. And, what's true of Staten Island should be true for Texas and Florida. I hope they, and anti-******* of all persuasions, survive in spite of their resistance. And if they do get sick, there will always be people to take care of them no matter what. What happened to yesterday's temp? It should have been 98.1 and I'm not sure why it didn't post other than the half carafe of red wine I had at dinner. temp today 98.6

Journal of the Plague Years, Day 395. I try to post about my own observations, and not re-hash what is on the news. But this week some potentially good news came out that is hard to ignore. The cdc came out with lots of guidelines on mask wearing and vaccines. There are charts that show fully vaccinated people have can leave off masks if with other vaccinated people when outdoors except in large packed crowds. non-vaccinated still have to wear masks in many cases. indoors everyone should be wearing masks due to the risk of becoming a carrier from someone else, even if you don't get sick. I don't know if simple guidelines will convince anti-v****** that now is the time to get their shots. but most of this loosening up is for outdoor activity. down here in The Village I think we are probably as well vaccinated as any non-institutionalized population so as I wander lower Manhattan this weekend I'll try and notice if masks are less prevalent or about the same. It's a good step, hope it convinces people. temp today 98.0

Journal of the Plague Years, Day 398, Monday May 3. (my mom's birthday, she would be 107) This weekend I tried to see if the recent changes in cdc recommendations about masks have made a difference. I couldn't tell for sure. Without doing a literal nose count it seemed that the slight majority of people walking around in the Village didn't have masks, but the slight majority of people down in Chinatown did. It was impossible to count accurately and see if Asian Americans vs non-Asians whites had a different profile but I couldn't tell. One thing seems sure, the cdc guidelines about walking in the open didn't make a tremendous difference. There are still a lot of people with masks, being careful, and it's also not possible to know who of the masked vs maskless had their vaccines. People are just being careful. That's ok, a little extra caution is good and wearing a face mask is not a tremendous burden. temp today 97.9

Journal of the Plague Years, Day 399. Yesterday I posted about what people appear to be doing now that the cdc has changed guidelines for mask wearing. Today, what I've been doing. Basically, I still wearing my mask out in public all the time. It's not that big a burden and I've gotten used to it. Since I'm fully vaccinated, the chances of me catching the virus out in public, let alone getting sick from it, are infinitely small. But, if by some freak chance I do get "colonized" (that's the term when an infection is somewhere in your system but doesn't give you symptoms) it will be a real problem. By DOH rules, I get tested for covid at my office every week. If I am colonized and test positive for any reason, I'm supposed to be away from the office, the facility, and my patients for two weeks. I'm not set up for, nor do I want, "remote" visits with my patients. My visits are in person, nothing remote. So, I wear the mask, at least for now. temp today 98.8

Journal of the Plague Years, Day 400. Walking back home yesterday, at about 5:30, I passed Chelsea Market and decided to go in. I was shocked. The guards at the doors enforced mask wearing for everyone. Inside, the place was really, really empty. I expected it to be a little empty but at least half of the stores were closed and only a few people were walking the main hallway. Those places that were open usually had a few customers. Even Los Tacos No. 1 which is always packed had only one or two people. Only the Lobster Place and an Asian restaurant next to it had more than a half dozen people sitting and having dinner. Outside, on 15th street, at least three restaurants with curbside tables had at least a dozen diners each. The nice warm sunny weather may have pulled people from the dark inside to the bright outside, but there still weren't a lot, especially when Hudson street usually had much bigger crowds at the same time. I don't know how these places will survive, if they get crowded on the weekends to make up for Tuesday night emptiness or what. I hope the Chelsea Market managers, whoever they are, give these places really good deals on their rents. I never thought I would miss the Chelsea Market crowds that kept so many of the attractive eating places out of reach because of long lines, but I did miss the people. When I go to my favorite opened restaurants, I'm really happy when I have a hard time finding a seat. Their crowding will help them survive. Chelsea Markets stores? Who knows? temp today 97.6

Journal of the Plague Years, Day 401. The department of health, the DOH, has made public some new data on covid vaccinations. There is now a website where the vaccination rates for both nursing home and assisted living facilities showing staff and resident rates. The site is: https://covid19vaccine.health.ny.gov/federal-long-term.... My facility has about 95% for residents and about 75% for staff, which puts us in the middle of the pact. Part of this is for transparency but sometimes data are misleading and might be a little out of date. The rates of immunization might not actually reflect the care at the facility, nursing home or ALF, which depends on many factors, like overall staffing or services available. But, what else might they do with this information? Right now, rules for nursing homes or ALFs cover the entire field as a whole. It might be that individual data might enable the state to modify rules based on each individual facility so highly vaccinated facilities might have more liberal regulations. We'll see. temp today 98.0

Journal of the Plague Years, Day 402. As usual, I'm looking for something upbeat for a Friday post. Not much dramatically better has happened this week, except for one thing. Bars are reopening. I won't get a chance to examine the effects of this change until the weekend, and maybe not then if the rainy weather keeps me indoors away for the bars/restaurants effected. But, some of my weekends travels usually take me past, and sometimes into, various bars in lower Manhattan. Whether these newly opened places are attractive, or even nostalgic, enough to pull people inside from the sidewalk tables we've gotten used to is an open question. I'll let you know next week what I find. And remember, if I'm hung-over on Monday night when I do my first post it's all because of my dedication in bringing you all the freshest covid news on FB. temp today 98.2

Journal of the Plague Years, Day 405, Monday May 10. Walking around on a chilly and rainy Saturday, I did my best to see what is happening with newly opened bars, and ongoing inside and outside dining. At about 4-5 along downtown restaurant/bar heavy streets I noticed a few things. In those places that had bars, inside and outside dining, most bars only had a few people sitting there, but the outside tables were still pretty full in spite of the weather. Inside dining was a little more crowded than the bars, but not much. In other words outside dining trumps inside dining and inside dining trumps bars (sorry for the repeated use of the T word). Those places with only bar space and no outside tables, had pretty full bar seats, maybe even beyond the social distancing guidelines. I don't know if this will continue when weather gets hot and humid or will people be driven inside for the air conditioning, social distancing or not. One owner was thinking of getting fans for the outside tables, at least for the moderately hot days. Those facers reading this who live downtown or who are near similar establishments can let me know if this priority ranking is occurring in other places. As much as I might like to, I couldn't really do bar hopping to get an inside view or I would have been in a coma by the end of the day and I've knelt in front of the porcelain God enough times in my life already. temp today 98.0

Journal of the Plague Years, Day 406. There has been a lot of talk about increased violence in the subways, and lots of newspaper and TV news reports on these crimes. What have I seen? For sure, there are people in the subways who exhibit bizarre behavior and appear to have mental health problems, although I have never seen an actual crime. What I have seen is a big increase in cops since the stabbing of four people about a month ago, with the death of two of them. 500 cops were assigned to the subways, where there had hardly been any before that, and I've posted about them recently. Last Friday, coming home at about 5 PM, the 2/3 subway lines have 5 stops before I'm home. Although I wasn't looking for them, I saw cops on the station platforms of 3 of the 5 stations. There may even have been cops on the other stations I didn't see. And, there were a lot of them. Today, only cops on one station. I don't know if this increase has cut crime in the last month, it might be too early to tell. But, there definitely is a change in the atmosphere down there. We'll see if this makes a difference. If crime drops, the police department will brag about it, and if it doesn't the department will be criticized. There are plenty of people running for mayor on both sides of the "more cops vs defund the cops" debate and so plenty of supporters and critics are waiting in the wings, and in front of the TV cameras for the results to come in. We'll see. temp today 98.1

Journal of the Plague Years, Day 407. I posted about my experiences on the subways, but today one of the nurses I work with described hers. She is on the evening shift and leaves work at 11:30 to midnight to ride the same 2 and 3 Seventh Avenue express that I ride at 5. The first car she went into had a guy smoking pot. The smoke was so much that she moved to the next care where there were four homeless people and her. She didn't feel safe so moved to the next car where she finally was able to sit safely (relatively). Late night closing of the subways has made them cleaner during the day, but there are still plenty of homeless who use it at night. I asked her if this happens all the time and she said yes, although not exactly the same way. Plenty of homeless at night. But then she shrugged her shoulders and proudly said, in a thick Haitian accent, "Well, I'm a New Yorker." temp today 98.2

Journal of the Plague Years, Day 408. When I walk home from my office or some other place, like my savings bank, I try to take different routes so I won't get bored seeing the exact same sites every time. Last night I walked down 10th avenue into the Meatpacking district. I was happy to see that the Brass Monkey bar in the middle of Meatpacking, was open. It's a large place with two stories of large bars and a roof top restaurant. The bars were almost completely empty, but the roof top had 5-10 people. I stopped there in the sun, had a Guiness, and enjoyed the view of a beautiful sunset over the Hudson and New Jersey (the state of my birth in Newark). The emptiness was a little depressing, but since this is such a large place with, presumably, a very large overhead, I expected it to be completely closed. Even a weakly opened establishment still illustrates hope. There haven't started their packed Friday night happy hours yet, but the fact that they're still there is a hopeful sign. Maybe a few more months, with more customers and less masks (legally) and things will be close to normal and I can resume dropping in on Friday evenings for a Guiness or two and some really tasty bar food. We'll see. temp today 98.4

Journal of the Plague Years, Day 409. What is there to be hopeful about? The cdc loosens guidelines on masks was good. Slow decrease in new cases, nationally, is also good. I'm looking more locally. The ALF where I work used to be 100% occupied with several month waiting list. Now, with covid, we are 20% empty. But things are picking up. I used to get 2-3 new admissions a month with 1 or 2 coming back from rehab. This last week I've had about 4-5 new admissions and several people back from rehab. Logically, only one good week does not make a trend. But when you're trying to be hopeful in what is still a dire situation, in spite of good news from cdc, you try to predict trends at a very early stage. There seems to be an uptick in new admissions over the next few weeks also. Our place offers a wide variety of services and accepts people on Medicaid (besides being in a prime location on 5th avenue in Manhattan which is why we used to be 100% with a waiting list.) I'm hoping we can go back to this. By the way, it's a non-profit community run place, so I don't have any financial investment in it. Only 17.5 years there doing primary care. (look up Vistaon5th.org) temp today 98.6

Journal of the Plague Years, Day 412, Monday May 17. The cdc set out guidelines for mask wearing and it seems that people who have been vaccinated have a lot more leeway. Only indoors where there are large crowds and minimal social distancing should we were masks. How about small crowds? I was sitting on a bench on Hudson street this morning having my bacon/egg/cheese sandwich and a coffee. It is right in front of the local post office. It opened about 10:15 with 8-10 people in line. There was a little social distancing, although I couldn't see if it was exactly 6 feet.

Over the course of the next 20 minutes about another dozen people came and stood in line waiting to go in. Every person was wearing a mask both on line and when entering. Some of these people may have been vaccinated but they were masked anyway. I don't know if a small post office is what the cdc had in mind for a "crowd". As I posted recently about myself, I were a mask a lot more than I have to, just to be safe. It looks like there twenty or so people were doing the same. Things are getting better, but just a little more caution, especially about something as easy to do as wear a mask, seems to appeal to a lot of people. temp today 98.1

Journal of the Plague Years, Day 413. There has been a very small change in Medicare rules that indicate a new approach to the use of rehabilitation. Usually, if a person goes into a hospital and stays for three nights, he or she can then go to a rehab facility and Medicare will pay for it, sometimes up to a few months. Sometimes this is the only way to get Medicare to pay. Recently, the rules have changed so that only 2 days in the hospital are needed. This doesn't look like a lot since you end up in rehab anyway, but it does do two things. It takes pressure off the hospital and might save Medicare money since rehab is cheaper than hospital days. One of the controversies early in the epidemic was the transfer of covid positive patients from the hospital back to nursing homes, where many died. Although the care in the nursing home for any one patient would not be a thorough as care in the hospital, the hospitals were collapsing under the strain. These transfers helped the hospitals open up How many transfers who died in the nursing homes might have stayed alive in the hospital had to be balanced with how many more would die in the hospital if they were overwhelmed. Relaxing the three day rule continues to help the hospitals and gets people to rehab, where they might be safer anyway. I've had patients admitted to the hospital when it was clear that they needed rehab and the three day rule ways frequently a time and money waster. After this is over someone will have to research whether the hospitals and their patients were helped more than the transfers were hurt. temp today 97.9

Journal of the Plague Years, Day 414. Walking from my office to the subway this afternoon, I passed a sign for covid testing at a little curbside site. It was, I think labelled "testQ covid testing" or something like that. I have seen these pop-up mobile testing units around but didn't give them much thought. I couldn't find this company, or organization, on the internet but I found lots and lots of place that do covid testing. Not vaccines, testing. A while back I posted about lines in front of CityMD offices when they were the only ones doing testing. I'm not sure why so many are getting tested now. Are they vaccinated and want to see if they are infected in spite of the vaccine? Are they unvaccinated and hope that a lot of negative tests will give them an excuse not to get it? Are they symptomatic or not? I don't know the motivation but there are plenty of places doing it so there must be some demand. Although testing availability and motivation is interesting it doesn't change the most important thing. We still have to get everyone vaccinated no matter how the tests ae going. temp today 98.6

Journal of the Plague Years, Day 415. Yesterday I posted about a curbside covid tester called testQ and how I didn't know who they were or what they were doing. Today I took a closer look and they are actually called labQ (labq.com) and there work is much clearer. TGhey might be independent but they have some type of affiliation with Mt. Sinai. Besides testing they are also involved in some type of program to encourage covid survivors to donate plasma for the treatment of others. They also advertise other testing sites which are Sinai affiliated hospitals in Brooklyn, although they don't mention the curbside mobile sites. In either case they are advertising programs, whether testing or plasma acquisition, which appear to be beneficial. Why people are getting these tests is still unclear, but there wasn't a line in front of this mobile site yesterday or today, like there was in front of the CityMD offices a few months ago, so the overall demand for tests might be decreasing. If this will continue or will covid testing be routinely done in doctor's offices in the future, I don't know. We'll see. 98.0

Journal of the Plague Years, Day 416. A while back I posted about how this has been a very, very mild flu season. At the start of covid doctors, including myself, were worried that covid and flu were going to be added to each other and increase problems. But, flu cases have actually dropped to only a few percent of what they normally are. Covid and flu are not the only respiratory viruses, there are hundreds, if not thousands, of them. This involves me personally. When I lived in Los Angeles from 88 to 90 I never got a cold or sinus infection during the winter. When I moved back to NYC I started to get 2-3 sinus infections and 2-3 mild colds every Winter. Sometimes I needed antibiotics, sometimes just a strong cough syrup, both of which I can prescribe for myself (it's good to be the doctor!). This winter, nothing. Not one cold. Not one sinus infection. No antibiotics. No cough syrup (I'll miss it). One person having a good winter for just one year is not exactly a scientific sample. But it's consistent with the national flu data. So, maybe the NPIs, non-pharmacological interventions (masks, isolation, hand washing, testing and tracing) might actually be something we may want to use again during normal times. Before covid I remember seeing pictures of Japanese and I think Koreans wearing masks when out in public during Winter months. I used to think this was gross over-reaction. Maybe not. temp today 97.7

Journal of the Plague Years, Day 419, Monday May 17th. Today is an update on a previous theme. Last week, at about 4:30 when I went to the 110th St. subway there were TEN cops there. Four on the street at the top of the stairs, two near the turnstile, and four on the platform. Several of the cops were writing out something, maybe a summons, for a young black guy but there was no argument and I didn't get close enough to see exactly what they were doing. I didn't post this late last week since I didn't know if this was a good sign or a bad one. Is is good that there are plenty of cops in the subways to keep us safe. Or are things in the subways so dangerous that an army of cops are needed. Every week it seems that more are added, either a few hundred MTA or city cops. There is still plenty of violence in the subway which is picked up and amplified by the media, but there's plenty of violence on the streets also. I don't know if covid decreasing will take the pressure off people, including mentally ill or criminally inclined ones, and decrease crime, or if these trends will increase. By the way, I seldom see cops on the train, but almost always at the stations. We'll see what happens, if I live long enough to post about it. temp today. 98.3

Journal of the Plague Years, Day 420. Oops, yesterday I gave the date as May 17 instead of May 24. That's what happens when you post late at night after a 2.5 hour Zoom meeting. Today, when walking to the subway to go home, there were two blue canopies at the corner of 110th and Lenox Avenue. There were a few people there giving out vaccines, but no ID as to who was running it. I asked one of the staff who they were and they said they were from Columbia, giving free vaccines to people walking by. When I asked how it was going they said they got a good response when they told anyone who stopped to ask that the vaccine was free and there was a $50 stipend for people getting the vaccine. I hadn't heard of this program, from Columbia or anyone else, and I don't know all the details. They were busy and I didn't want to distract them too much. But it seemed like this was a simple, no strings attached, way of getting people to take the shots. They said they moved around from day to day and I'm not sure where they will be tomorrow, but this was an interesting, although somewhat mysterious program to get people vaccinated. I couldn't find the program on the internet, and they didn't even have their tents with identification, but they were giving free shots. If anybody finds details about this let me know. Whoever is running the program should get some acknowledgement for their good deed. temp today 98.7

Journal of the Plague Years, Day 421. Like old man river, NYC keeps rolling on regardless of immediate events, even a disaster like covid. Parallel to the covid events of the last year or so, the city has been doing other things unrelated to the plague. One of these is the re-emergence of The Village Voice. Old timers will know that it started in 1955 as the country's first alternative news paper, but one with national prominence because of the writers (Norman Mailer, Nat Hentoff, Wayne Barrett and so many others) and the ground breaking coverage of politics, culture, arts, and lifestyle, especially the gay community. A few years ago it stopped the print edition, then I think it stopped the website. But now it's back. The issue I saw is the Spring issue, vol LXIII, No 1. entitled "New York's Coming Back and So Are We." which is given away free someplace or other in the city (I got my copy in the recycling room of my building). It has current political events, entertainment, movie reviews by Michael Musto, along with articles from years ago. The Voice didn't disappear because of covid and probably hasn't come back because of it. But, the city, The Voice, and much more will keep rolling along when covid is just a distant ugly memory. temp today 98.3

Journal of the Plague Years, Day 422. On Day 420 I posted about a mysterious blue canopy with people giving vaccines. They were back today but now with identification. They are with something called the COMPASS study (Community Prevalence of SARs cov-2, at compass-study.org) which is a national study trying to determine covid prevalence in communities around the country. Several government agencies, public health organizations, and networks used for other epidemiology studies like AIDs support organizations. 58,000 people will be enrolled at a dozen sites in the country. The format is to collect blood samples to see who had covid previously, do a swab test, and maybe even give vaccines although that might not be available at all sites. At this on one 110th street and Lenox avenue they were collecting this info and giving vaccines. They had a few staff members and about 10 people who got the vaccine or were giving info.

Participants in the study can't ask to be in or make appointments. The staff under the canopy ask people walking by if they would like to participate. It's entirely random. They are also trying to find out about racial differences in vaccinations and infections. This looks a lot more substantial than a few days ago. Keep this in mind if the study ever hits the mainline media. You heard it here first. temp today 98.6

Journal of the Plague Years, Day 423. (A little late) On the theme of NYC rolling on in spite of every immediate disaster, like covid, here's another. The opening of Little Island park in the Hudson river, aka Diller's island (littleisland.org) shows that some things keep getting done. Although it was controversial at the start, required a few hundred million dollars and more to come later, intervention by the governor, and several years of work, it eventually got done. I walked around it at 11 AM on Sunday when it was sunny and warm. It was packed. The park is cute with lots of areas to hang out in sequestered from the rest of the park, two performance areas, a food court and bathrooms (!), and lots of nice views inward toward Manhattan and across the river to Jersey. I don't know how crowded it will get. When more tourists discover it, maybe as crowded as the Highline. If the weather is poor and the cold winds blow in from the river, maybe a little empty. Performances will start as covid declines. There are lots of pictures on their website along with those posted by other Facers on the public screens of this Facebook site. But if it gets too crowded, remember the words of Yogi Berra. "Nobody goes there anymore, it's much too crowded." 98.5

Journal of the Plague Years, Day 427, June 1. A lot of the empty storefronts are being put to use by spreading art work. A program called artontheavenyc.com is putting artists works in storefronts around the Village. About twenty local businesses are supporting it and about a dozen storefronts have the paintings in their windows. some of the stores are functioning normally like the Lortel theater on Christopher street and Contessa hair cutters on Hudson. But most appear closed, although I haven't gone to every address to confirm it. The program last until July so look at the website or if you're in the area look at the windows. There are also QR codes, but I could only get the one on the main poster to work right. I don't know if this program is entirely due to covid caused empty storefronts, but it seems to be taking advantage of the situation. And their website has some information about new applications, so some form of this program might be extended beyond June. An appropriate response to the epidemic in art filled Greenwich Village. temp today 98.3

Journal of the Plague Years, Day 428. I've talked about cops on the subway before, but from a distance. Today it got closer. I got on the first car of a 2 train at about 5 PM with a half dozen people scattered around the car. I was in the back of the car but I heard some people at the front arguing. From the voices there were two women and maybe a guy adding in, with profanities all around. I didn't turn and look since I didn't want to break two subway rules: never look directly at people acting badly and never make eye contract with people, any people. After the arguing died down one of the people started to play really loud music, some type of Motown rhythm and blues tune that would have been nice someplace else. The conductor announced the train was being held up by the dispatcher, a routine announcement, and then "NYPD to the first car". Over the next few minutes he said it a few times. Just before 96th street five cops walked into the car, four near the door and one at the front talking to the conductor in his booth. At 96th, three of the cops went over to one of the women and asked her to get off, which she wasn't doing. She wasn't acting strange at that time, but got off the train and was speaking to the cops peacefully on the platform as the train pulled out. No fighting, no arguing, no gunshots, etc. Pretty anti-climactic, fortunately. I hope everything during my subway trips stays at this level. temp today 98.8

Journal of the Plague Years, Day 429. A day or two ago Mayor D******* and councilwoman Margaret Chin announced that the senior centers all over the city are opening up again. This is good for socialization and quality of life for older adults, 65 and above. But during their discussion they mentioned at a full 74% of old adults are immunized. 74%?! Are these people crazy? the Daily News verified this with a figure of 72% with at least one shot and 65% with both shots. Young folks who think they are immune are getting lower shots, as are the staff members of my facility (60% at first, 75% now). But older people have no excuse. They know they can get sick, they know they can die. Why only 75%? I don't know, but I hope they smarten up before too many realize they made a serious mistake. Fauci has said that just about everyone without a vaccine will eventually get covid. Some will die. Just about nobody with the vaccine will die. Incentives like lottery tickets, free beer, etc will help but what will it take? temp today 98.8

Journal of the Plague Years, Day 430. A while back I mourned the passing of four of my favorite places. Here's an update. Sweet Corner pastry shop has been replaced with Lucky Louie's fried chicken place. The chicken is good, but I haven't seen big crowds, so who knows if it will survive. Westville on 10th street has been replaced with a sushi restaurant. Philip Marie is still empty but there is construction going on there with new tile steps going in and the inside is gutted. I don't know if the landlord is doing this to make it marketable or if a new place is already coming in. The fourth, Bethel Gourmet foods on Greenwich Avenue across from St. Vincent's triangle is still empty, but I would guess it has a really high rent because of location. So, two or maybe three places are bouncing back out of four. Without covid, food places have always been very competitive with high turnover, so I don't know what will happen to these places. But at least for now, people are fighting back demonstrating resiliency. Am I using the word "resiliency" too much on these posts? Well, it just seems appropriate and I hope I can keep using it as the city wakes up. temp today 98.7

Journal of the Plague Years, Day 431, Monday June 7. I've posted recently that I've seen lots of cops on the subways, scattered around at various stations. The station nearest my office is at 110th street and Central Park North, on the 2 and 3 Seventh Avenue express lines. Friday I saw something there I've never seen at any of the stations. There was a white shirt officer there. These are the senior supervising officers that oversee the blue uniformed ones. You see them sometimes at parades or demonstrations, but I've never seen one on the subway. Is it because crime is higher or because more cops need more supervision. It might also be because 110th and CP North is a somewhat special station. More on this tomorrow. temp today 96.9

Journal of the Plague Years, Day 432. Follow up. The 2/3 station at 110th and Central Park North is small. No connections to other subways, although bus lines on the surface. It mostly serves the local neighborhood and during rush hours there usually isn't a big crowd. But, the platform is in the middle of the station with the uptown and downtown trains on the sides of the platform, not on opposite sides of the tracks like other stops. Cops there can react to both uptown and downtown headed trains. There's a lot to react to. The end of March 2020 a homeless guy set a fire at the station and in the evacuation an MTA employee, Garrett Goble, died. Another time a mental ill man who was naked and bothering people on the station pushed somebody onto the tracks, and went down there to prevent him from getting back on the platform. The ill man accidentally touched the third rail, and died. There have been various fights and slashings, recently two slashings within a few hours of each other. For a small station, it has a lot of dangerous action. And, if I could notice it, I'm sure the cops did also. temp today 98.2

Journal of the Plague Years, Day 433. I was going to move on from the subway, but I saw something today I need to document. At the 110th street station, likened by some to a third word ambiance, I saw a man walking the station. Like old people walking the malls, this guy was old, bald, white, hunched over a little, with a t-shirt and shorts, marching back and forth over the 2 block length of the station with a determined look and a pretty quick pace. While I was there he made three complete laps up and down the platform, and I don't know how many before I got there. He wasn't waiting for a train since he left the station before any trains came. It made sense to fast walk underground which wasn't quite as hot as the street, and which also, again, had a few cops there. I don't know if this has anything to do with covid, since he was maskless in spite of huffing and puffing as he did his rounds. If you see or hear of anyone else doing this anywhere else, remember you heard it here first, as far as I know. temp today 98.7

Journal of the Plague Years, Day 434. Two nights ago I went to my first indoor concert in the last year. The Washington Square Music Festival has four outdoor concerts each year in Washington Square Park in The Village. This Tuesday is was rained out and we met in the Judson Memorial Church facing the park. In a room designed for 200 people, about 75 well spaced out (spatially not mentally) people listened to a concert of music by the Harlem Chamber Players. It was mostly classical music with one gospel piece, "He's got the whole world in his hands", appropriate for a church venue. The performance was great, the soprano was great and it was the first indoor get together that I can remember. I think most people wore their masks, as did I, for most of the performance. I saw several friends in person (!) not via zoom or Facebook. One more step for normalcy. temp today 98.0

Journal of the Plague Years, Day 435. Last weekend I was walking down Christopher street to my bagel connection and a large part of the intersection of it with Bleeker street had a large green lawn set up on it and a lot of Bleeker closed to traffic. A few people were doing yoga, but not much going on. Later in the afternoon I passed again and there was a crowd of a few dozen, a performer singing and strumming a guitar and a big sign reading "Shop the Village". I looked it up (shopthevillage.nyc) and it seems that about 40 village stores, many of them competitors in normal times, had set up a program on June weekends for musical performances, food pop-ups, children's activities, etc, around Greenwich Village to encourage people to come out and patronize local businesses, mostly for eating or clothes shopping. The fighting that local businesses to stay open during covid hasn't just been by individuals, but it looks like they've banded together. It seems like a good idea, hope it takes off. I'll do my part, back to the bagel shop. temp today 98.7

Journal of the Plague Years, Day 438, Monday June 14. I think there will be a lot of good news this week. Here's the first. I thought as covid waned bars and restaurants who just got by would get back to their pre-covid status. I didn't foresee that some places would use the opportunity of low rents and empty storefronts to actually expand, and not just survive. Around the corner from me, the Austrian restaurant Wallsee has been there for years and has survived covid. They also just took over an empty neighboring storefront next door which they have appropriately called "Wallsee Next Door". L'Artusi, an Italian restaurant on Tenth street also has been around a while and has survived. But they also took over a corner spot on Hudson and Tenth and are opening "B'Artusi" and possibly another place next to that called La Porta. I guess any place that was determined to survive, and who has deep pockets to expand, shouldn't just be satisfied with the status quo. These places are just a few blocks from my house, but they can't be the only places jumping on this opportunity. Any Facers reading this who know of other places that are expanding, please post and let us know. The more positive news the better. temp today 98.5

Journal of the Plague Years, Day 439. Good news from the ALF where I work. The state no longer requires we test every staff member every week. It has been a real pain doing this. The two RNs who do the swabbing are also our two highest clinical administrators and they have lots of other important things to do. The library is unusable since it is packed with supplies for testing. And, it's a nuisance. A few mild cases among the staff were picked up months ago, but none recently for quite a while. Now the state says we should swab staff, and probably patients, only when symptomatic. Although there is always a case that can slip by undetected, with 96% of residents and now about 75% staff fully vaccinated, the chance of major spread is less. If city numbers start to get bad again because of some new mutant flying in from India, or wherever, then this will change. But the DOH has been very hard nosed with requirements and I'll give them the benefit of the doubt that this is a good move. More good news over the next few days. temp today 98.9

Journal of the Plague Years, Day 440. More good news. The nightly movies are back at the ALF. Because group meetings are now allowed we can resume movies every night at the facility. Current movies from Netflix, or maybe some old classics, are shown every night with maybe one or two dozen people watching. This is only a fraction of the hundred people living there but it's a start. We are trying to break the hermit-like behavior that many residents have fallen into. The state, and ALFs themselves, are trying to preserve independent among the residents and sitting in your room alone watching TV or the computer screen doesn't do it. People get physically deconditioned and sometimes mentally deconditioned (depressed/anxious/isolated). More activities to get people active tomorrow. temp today 97.9

Journal of the Plague Years, Day 441. Yet more good news. The dining room is slowly opening up. While on quarantine, residents still needed to get 3 meals a day. These were delivered to each person in each apartment for each meal. Sometimes they were eaten and sometimes wasted. Now everyone is invited one day a week for two meals, lunch and dinner. Also, there is a walk in option for people not scheduled on that day but there are a few extra tables and people can just walk in for extra meals instead of waiting in their rooms. Residents have gotten used to room service and this isn't good for them. Social isolation, physical debility and increased depression and anxiety all seem to have increased over the year. Just walking to the dining room helps with socialization. In the dining room residents seem to eat more of their meals and they can be monitored by dining room staff so that those who don't eat will be detected quickly. All this is good. Hope it can increase until everyone is up there three times a day every day. We're slowly inching toward that day. temp today 97.6

Journal of the Plague Years, Day 442. After all the relatively good, although minor, news I've outlined this week, I've realized there is something more significant that might be happening. Previously I've posted about the drop in flu cases this year, possibly as much as 99%. I've also mentioned that I haven't gotten any of my 3-6 respiratory infections this winter. It turns out, this is a very wide phenomenon. Several staff at my ALF who get colds every winter said they had nothing this year. My own physician said he saw almost no respiratory cases this year although this was the peak winter season. I realized that the same is true with my practice. Every winter for about 3-4 months I see patients with congestion, runny noses, colds, coughs, bronchitis attacks, sinus infections, and even a few pneumonias. Usually 1-3 cases every day. This year, nothing. I can't remember the last time I prescribed claritin or cough syrup although I prescribe a ton of it every year. And these infections would have occurred just before the covid vaccines came out, so they aren't responsible for the good news. Only NPIs (non-pharmacological interventions of hand washing, isolation, social distancing, masks, etc) were available. But the results were great. Next winter people aren't going to put up with these restrictions all winter like they did this last year. But maybe a few of the items like masks, frequent temperature taking, isolation for those with symptoms (especially coughs) etc might be acceptable to patients even without the threat of another epidemic. I hope we all remember these facts next winter. temp today 98.5

Journal of the Plague Years, Day 445, Monday June 21. Stuff has been happening in The Village that may or may not be covid related. There have been a lot of late night parties in Washington Square

Park recently with partiers and local residents arguing with each other. Lots of late night music/noise until 2 or 3 in the morning.. Lots of this is in the media, on YouTube, or locally on the internet (thevillagesun.com). There have always been lots of music, partying and drug use in the park, alternating with police crack downs, but recently it's been a lot more, bigger crowds and more amplified sound. Covid? Some say that being cramped up for a year has made people more likely to bust loose more than in previous years. I don't know which is right, but now some violence and possible problems with mental health behavior has started to surface. It's a little like the Seattle Automatous Zone last year. I just hope they figure out what to do before someone gets killed, like in Seattle. If it's covid maybe as the rest of the city opens people will find other, safer, places to party. temp today 98.4

Journal of the Plague Years, Day 446. Very negative post yesterday, but very good one today. Over the weekend, while having pastry at Cafe Palermo on Mulberry Street, I heard a rumor that the cancelled San Gennaro festival was being reinstated and will be held this September. I check their website and it looks like it's true. I've been going to San Gennaro almost every year for the last fifty years or so, since I was in my twenties. It's a very New York tradition with lots of food, crowds, shadey games of chance and NYC atmosphere, in honor of a patron saint of Naples. Some can't stand it because of the crowds ("I hate this fucking feast. You can't walk around in your own neighborhood." Robert DeNiro as Johnny Boy in Mean Streets, 1973). But, if you can tolerate that, or come at a less crowded time, you can get overpriced sausage sandwiches to your hearts content. Something to look forward to for September, unless we have a relapse. temp today 97.4

Addendum. Oops, forgot. When you hear about this remember you heard it here first. If I'm wrong forget I ever mentioned it.

Journal of the Plague Years, Day 447. Today's post will seem trivial, but it's a baby step in the right direction. Today I wore a tie to work.

No big deal, normally. But I haven't worn a tie during the entire covid lock down. It's not just because I hate wearing a tie, which I do, but because it is just one more surface that can be contaminated with virus particles. Some of my patients might like the formal appearance of a doctor in a tie, but I try to be as informal as possible for the patients who are already nervous about seeing a doctor. I won't be doing this every day, at least not yet, but it's one tiny step toward normal behavior, or at least toward pre-covid behavior. 98.1

Journal of the Plague Years, Day 448. I've wondered about how the restaurants and bars that have survived this last year accomplished it. I figured that landlords, rather than have an empty storefront at a time when they couldn't find a new renter, would give businesses a break. In my totally unscientific survey of three businesses I found one where the pastry shop owner owned the building, so he could do anything he wanted with his own place. In another place, a bar/restaurant, the landlord cut a deal and gave the place a break. In the third, a restaurant, the landlord is being inflexible and now wants back rent in full. All three of these places survived, and all are doing good business right now. I don't know if there are any lessons from this divergent pattern or even if three places is actually a meaningful pattern. But, I'll ask around, and I hope other Facers reading this do the same, and let's figure out how part of this city actually survived. Just in case this happens again in our lifetime. temp today 98.5

Journal of the Plague Years, Day 449. More news of NYC bounce back. A few years ago a large restaurant on Bleeker street closed. I think it was called Manahatta and it had a Greek diner type menu. After being closed for years, this weekend I saw work on it with a sign saying "Uncle Theo's will open soon." Trigger Thompson, a friend of ours in our posting group, is opening three ice cream places in Manhattan on Delancey and Division streets and St. Mark's Place. These new places might have nothing to do with Covid but they do indicate coming back to normal. Normal means lots of bars and restaurants and lots of turnover. But coming back to that also means coming back in general. When there are so many doom and gloom articles about how NYC is dead and won't recover because office work is now remote, it's good to get alternative facts. Thomas Huxley was credited with the quote "there's nothing so sad as a beautiful theory slain by an ugly fact." There new openings turn that around and now an ugly theory is being slain by some beautiful, or at least tasty, facts. At least, I hope so. temp today 98.2

Journal of the Plague Years, Day 452, Monday June 28. Recently I posted about a neighborhood effect to get people to shop in Greenwich Village. It is called Shop the Village. I passed by some people gathered to hear music on one of the blocked off streets, and I've seen more of their decals on sidewalks. Tonight I heard from a few people who took a closer look than I did. One weekend the events were empty, and on another, when there was music, there seemed to be a good crowd listening. But both my friends agreed that people were not actually going into the stores. The events, and others around the neighborhood that I'm not aware of, had a mixed outcome, but actually increasing business might not be happening. Some of these experiments to recover from covid will be successful, and some won't. Right now the results for this particular attempt seem unclear or poor, but it goes until the middle of July I think. So, maybe it will kick in soon. But summer in Manhattan is often slow since people leave the city on various vacations. We'll see what happens. Anybody with more info, please chime in. (The ice cream place I mentioned last week is called Lucky Star ice cream, just to help them a little.) temp today 98.4

Journal of the Plague Years, Day 453. Trying to monitor openings and closings, I came across another source. A national website called Eater (ny.eater.com I think) has news of restaurants all over the country. A few days ago they had an announcement, which I can't find now, of B'Artusi and Via Porta opening on Hudson, which I also mentioned recently. I don't know who reported it first, but I'm glad to see others paying attention.

There's also The Village Sun and Westview News which has a column called "In and Out" talking about closings and openings. I've only looked at these in relationship to Lower Manhattan, especially the Village, and especially places that I can personally look at, and eventually eat in. More survival details soon. temp today 97.9

Journal of the Plague Years, Day 454. Why did some places close during covid and others fought to stay open? I only have a very small unscientific sample to use to examine this, but here it is. Several of the places that closed (Philip Marie, Golden Rabbit stationary, Bethel gourmet foods) had proprietors who I think were elderly and well within retirement age. Others that are staying open (Piccolo Angolo, Cafe Katja, Cafe Palermo) have owners who are roughly middle aged. So they all have several decades in the food business but are nowhere near retirement age. A very bad year like we just had might be enough to chase out newbies who are just getting into the food business along with those who have been doing it for 50 or so years, but not enough to chase out those who have invested a few decades already and have more decades to look forward to. In the course of a career in food there are all sorts of disasters that pop up (bankruptcies, stock market crashes, terrorist attacks, or maybe just an epic fire, or toxic Health Department or YELP review) and a really bad year can be just one more disaster to be dealt with. I don't know if this demographic reasoning is what is going on, especially when you consider how varied and individualistic restaurant owners are, but I'm just trying to make sense of what I see. Meanwhile, the best way to keep these places open is to patronize them. It's a fattening job, but somebody's got to do it! temp today 97.5

Journal of the Plague Years, Day 455 (a little late). Although mask wearing guidelines have loosened up recently, they are still required on the subways. Almost everyone complies with this, but there are always one or two who don't. I noticed something else, and started to count the maskless ones over the last few days. Of the twenty six completely maskless people, 23 were men and 3 were women. These weren't just homeless people and psychotics but people of all races and appearance. One generalization though, none were old. No gray haired men or women without a mask. And I didn't count those with mask who were wearing them wrong, because sometimes people, including myself, forget to pull up there masks to the proper position since we don't have to wear them above ground. There were just people who had no mask anywhere visible and who apparently had no intention of wearing one. Why are men so thick headed (in this particular case, not just in general)? Does going without a mask make them look butch? Are men more likely to be covid deniers? I don't know, but there it is. Another bit of strange behavior uncovered by the stress of the plague. temp today 98.1

Journal of the Plague Years, Day 456 (this was even later than usual, it is Friday's post). "Masks? Masks! We don't need no masks. We don't have to wear no stinkin masks!", a slight revision of a famous line from "The Treasure of Sierra Madre". So, out of overconfidence because they were vaccinated or just plain stubbornness a bunch of people, mostly men, refused to wear masks on the subways. That's the bad news. There's good news also. The vast majority of people in the subways or even above ground are wearing masks, and usually correctly. The cdc guidelines were criticized for being too complicated, but it seems that most people understood them well enough. Above ground there are few masks, and lots of people vaccinated. In subways and confined spaces, like small stores, people wear masks. And to show that this good news is more significant than the bad news, the new infection rate in NYC has plummeted to about 1%. As for the future, when the delta strain hits full force, I can only offer two words to the maskless and unvaccinated. Good luck. (you can insert whatever other two word greeting you would like, providing it won't get you kicked off FB.) temp today 98.5

Journal of the Plague Years, Day 460, Tuesday July 6. Irecently mentioned that the state is easing up on covid surveillence in assisted living. Today I was shown the actual letter from the state and it's a little more extensive than I thought. Not only has the weekly swab testing of staff been eliminated for asymptomatic staff, but even for outside vendors. Previously, if a repair person or even a cable installer or anyone coming into the facility didn't want to get tested/swabbed, the person wasn't allowed in. Some people coming in were refused entry because they refused the test. Now, both staff and outside vendors don't have to get swabbed. They do have to have their temperatures taken upon entry, just like you are supposed to do in a restaurant, but not the whole testing unless symptomatic. This helps a lot in getting help into the facility and relieves the administrative staff of a lot of work when they can be doing other things. It also gives the place an atmosphere of coming back to normal, which is psychologically beneficial to both staff and residents. temp today 97.2

Journal of the Plague Years, Day 461. There was a parade today in lower Manhattan, the Canyon of Heroes, where they have parades for note worthy people and events. The people being honored were those who kept the city going during covid. They included doctors, nurses, business owners, food deliverers, and countless other categories of people who had direct contact with the unvaccinated masses of people when the virus was sweeping the city and killing tens of thousands of people. It was very uplifting, the few parts I saw during my office hours. There were a few weak spots. EMT workers boycotted it because they haven't had a contract in about 3 years, and you can't pay the rent with parade ticker tape (although it's now confetti and not ticker tape). EMTs are part of the Fire Department and Fire Fighters unions also boycotted in solidarity with them. One news reported observed that the crowds observing the parade were a lot smaller than crowds that show up if a well known athlete or team are honored. Well, you take what you can get when you can get it. A parade is still a parade. I was at work but I was glad to see my colleagues participated and were honored. temp today 98.0

Journal of the Plague Years, Day 462 (a little late). There is another honor for first responders that is running into trouble. A memorial to them was to be set up in Battery Park, but local residents didn't want to give up the green space that would be eliminated so it was stopped. A letter to the Daily News, or maybe it was The Times, had a suggestion. Many responders, possibly the majority of them, were minorities, such as workers in long term care facilities, food workers, deliverers, etc, that maybe the monument should be in their communities. It suggested The Bronx or Brooklyn. Monuments often have two roles, to honor some group or individual and also to be in a central location so the public, including tourists, can come and visit. I have found what I believe is a perfect location. Tune in tomorrow (this post is getting too long) to find out where. temp today 98.3

Journal of the Plague Years, Day 463. The proposed memorial to first line workers was to be at Battery Park at the Southern end of NYC Council District 1. The Northern border is Houston street and I think there is a prime spot for a memorial there. At Houston and Christie streets starts Sara Roosevelt park, a massive public space with lots of playing fields, courts, and play grounds. It also has a large open plaza at the North end, bordering Houston. The surrounding neighborhood is, I believe, overwhelmingly minority and so this would be honoring those who comprised many of the first line workers (yesterday I forgot MTA workers who had scores of deaths). It would also attract tourists, local people, bridge and tunnel crowd, national and international tourists etc, because of it's location. It is within a few blocks of Yonah Shimmel's birthplace of the knish, Katz's deli, Orchard street, the Tenement museum and many more notable sites. It's also in an area packed with restaurants and bars and normally attracts all of these tourist groups. This is a very central location and just right for a memorial to an historical event like covid. temp today 98.7

Journal of the Plagues Years, Day 466, Monday July 12. Back to the subways. At the end of February a mentally ill person went through the subways and stabbed 4 people, killing two. There was such an outcry that there was a big increase in cops on the subways. I previously posted that before the stabbing you almost never saw cops in the subways. After that tragedy 500 additional cops were added, bringing the total to about 3000. A little later another 250 were added. Now you see cops all over the place. Virtually every day I see police on platforms or trains, sometimes in several stations. Crimes in the subways are frequently see on video cameras, on Youtube, in the papers (for those of us who still read newspapers). Documentation of crime has gone up a lot. But what is the result of all these cops? Tune in tomorrow. temp today 98.3

Journal of the Plague Years, Day 467. So what did all these cops accomplish? Assaults on the subways decreased by about 50% during the months of May and June. It's not clear if these were robberies, or assaults by people with mental health problems but the totals were down. Where did I get this data? FOX NEWS! For those who look for crime stories on Youtube, or TV, or the NY Post you know that the Fox system loves to publicize crime. Maybe it's because it attracts viewers/readers, or maybe because they can blame it on the D********, or maybe blame it on the race of the people involved. They revel in these stories. So when I saw this from Fox I was shocked. They are actually reporting good news on crime instead of fear mongering. Maybe this is so they can advocate for evens more cops. It certainly isn't to give credit to D******* or anyone in his administration. Tomorrow, how are the cops doing this? temp today 98.0

Journal of the Plague Years, Day 468. Yesterday morning on the uptown 2 train I saw three men without masks. One was carrying a fishing pole and got out at 110th street, probably to fish in the Harlem Meer a pond in the northeast corner of Central Park. As he left, still maskless, he passed six cops near the turnstile entrance who were talking to each other and didn't stop him or say anything. I found this really annoying and it seemed to me that they were taking a hands off approach, if they noticed him at all. Is this how they are operating? With all the police I've seen in the subway, only twice did I see them act. Once they seemed to be writing a ticket to a young guy and another time they took a women who was arguing with someone off the train. But maybe what appears to be a hands off approach is all you need. Just having a presence in the subways, on platforms, near turnstiles, or on trains, is all you need to deter at least some of the predators or mentally ill people from acting up. I don't know if a really aggressive approach, starting with the maskless ones, would work better or eventually produce some video documented confrontation that would undermine the entire process, and the initially good results. More stories, maybe with data, will have to come out and show what is working in the subways and what isn't. It's too big for me, but maybe eventually we'll will all figure it out together. temp today 98.1

Journal of the Plague Years, Day 469. I try not to use this post just to re-hash stuff in the mainline media, but there's something happening that's too big to ignore. Covid cases are increasing. In nyc there have been cases increasing from Staten Island to Hell's Kitchen and the total for NYC has increased over 1 % on average. The combination of delta mutant and non-vaxxers is doing this. Nationally, states with low vax scores are starting to increase although totals for the country are not in yet. We can't abolish the delta mutant, or whatever mutants come down the road in the future, but we can get vaccinated. There are lots of reasons not to get the vaccine, but every one is wrong. Just plain wrong. There's too much mis-information to answer every single one but over estimations of side effects, and conspiracy theories are two of the main ones. This is very bad news. But if we actually do get vaccinated the news will be very good. More on this tomorrow. temp today 97.2

Journal of the Plague Years, Day 470. The last case of polio I saw was in 1990. A Viet Namese refugee had it as a child and I was examining him for residual leg weakness many years later. The last case of chicken pox I saw was in 1985. I've never seen a case of diptheria, tetanus, mumps, or smallpox. The reason for all of these is the use of vaccines. They are effective and can actually wide out a disease. Why are anti-v****** not taking the vaccines? Some believe psychotic conspiracy theories like the vaccine containing micro chips or entering your DNA. Others worry about side effects. If all the medical side effects are true (Guillain Barre syndrome, myocarditis, endocarditis, etc) they are about 1/100,000 according to most recent data. You can get these same syndromes from catching actual covid at a rate of about 1/100, so that's a thousand times worse. And, covid can kill you. Many patients, friends and relatives who don't want the vaccine are taking other medications whose side effects are orders of magnitude more common and more serious than the vaccines, even if all the vaccine side effects turn out to be true. I just can't help get the feeling that some day I'll be going to the funeral of someone who died from covid because of vaccine fears. Excessive caution, skepticism, gulibility, or just plain stupidity shouldn't carry a death penalty. temp today 99.2

Journal of the Plague Years, Day 473, Monday July 19th. A few posts ago I mentioned how covid rates are moving up a little in NYC and maybe other places. I underestimated the problem by a wide margin. Now almost every state has an increase in covid rates, because of the delta strain and lack of vaccinations. Last year's experience would predict that in 1-2 months the big rise in cases will give a big rise in deaths. But, maybe not. Medical treatment for actual covid cases is a lot better now than last year with better ventilator use, ECMO treatments, monoclonal antibodies and maybe a few others. I hope these improvements work because getting people to take the vaccines isn't working very well. The Great Race of vaccines vs virus spread seems to be over with the virus winning. Now the race will be between the new delta virus and new treatments. Who will win that race is unclear. Check in a month or two. temp today 98.2

Journal of the Plague Years, Day 474. Yesterday I posted that the increase in covid cases might increase deaths and we should check in a month or two. I may have been wrong. There are some reports coming in about increased deaths. These are scattered and not confirmed by the cdc. But I learned that there is a reason for delays in statistics. It takes a week or two for the cdc to collect and collate death statistics from across the country and so death rates might be increasing already but we don't know it yet. These numbers are depressing, and maybe I'll have another day or two of bad news. But, there's good news too and I'll get to that by the end of the week. I promise (and I hope). temp today 98.8

Journal of the Plague Years, Day 475. I was planning to make today's post another downer and talk about the Beta strain (previously known as the South Africa strain) but I saw something today that changed my mind. Around my office at 108th and Fifth, and the subway at Lenox and 110th, I've occasionally seen young people with T-shirts that said "Test and Trace Corps". If I remember right, they sometimes had little tents and were doing covid testing. Today I saw a half dozen hanging around at 5 PM and I went over and asked them what they were about. It turns out that the NYC Dept of Health, through the Health and Hospitals Corporation (the City run hospitals) set up this program to do outreach into the community, Harlem in this case, to get more people to be tested or even to find a place to take the vaccine. They go out into the community, talk to people on the streets, give them literature, free masks, and the location of various sites for testing and vaccines. Response is mixed and goes from accepting to rejecting but not usually hostile. (Not many fanatic anti-v****** in Harlem?). They were mostly young, mostly minorities and all wearing their white "Test and Trace Corps" t-shirts. If you see any of them around other neighborhoods let me know. Let's spread the word since the virus isn't going to take a time out. temp today 98.5

Journal of the Plague Years, Day 476. The Test and Trace people yesterday pointed something out to me. I was speaking to them on Fifth Avenue and 109th street. A little bit into the block is the headquarters of the Common Pantry. They are a non-profit (I think) community group that gives food to individuals and organizations that need it. If you order from Fresh Direct, as I do, you know that you can click on an icon and donate anything from a single meal to a week of meals to go along with your order. I do this with every order I send in, usually about once every other week. They mentioned that Common Pantry is also arranging for vaccinations, and is one of the remaining spots in the neighborhood that offers them. They don't have too, as it's not part of their original mission, but they do. A Common Pantry volunteer who I spoke to while walking into work said she didn't know of the program, so either it's only done sporadically or it's so low key that their own people don't know about it. In any case, this seems like a pretty beneficial thing to be doing. If you order from Fresh Direct, please add on a Common Pantry meal option. If they're helping the community, we should be helping them. temp today 97.5

Journal of the Plague Years, Day 477. I've saved the best news for Friday. During the covid shut down, people have been quarantined in their rooms with medications and meals brought to them. This week, that stopped. They now have to come down to the Wellness Center (aka the medication room) to get their daily meds, unless they are competent enough to keep their meds in their rooms and be completely independent. About 3/4 residents come down. Also, they now have to go up to the beautiful dining room on the 14th floor with a spectacular view of Central Park, for all their meals. If they are too sick and immobile they can stay in their rooms, but there are only a few people like that. There are a few who are non-compliant and just refuse. But almost everyone complies with these rules/ It's better for their physical health as they are up and active and not getting weaker and deconditioned in their rooms. It's better for socialization and helps minimize depression and anxiety that people get from sitting in their rooms and looking at TV all day. Assisted living tries to maximize residents independence and keeping them active helps that a lot. This is a big post-covid improvement and step towards normalcy. temp today 96.8

Journal of the Plague Years, Day 280, Monday July 26. The city is having trouble getting its workers vaccinated. Too many are hesitant or anti-v******. At my assisted living, Vista on 5th, the state Medicaid program told us how to address this problem. All staff, whether vaccinated or not, have to wear masks. The residents don't have to right now. Earlier in the epidemic, all staff had to be tested twice a week, then eventually only once a week even if vaccinated. It was a pain logistically, but was done. Residents had voluntary testing and about 50% took it. I don't know if all city workers, or even the ones in hospitals, have to wear a mask whenever indoors and certainly with any patient contact. But to require masks and weekly tests is a first step to getting city workers to do this, or if they don't do it they will at least be minimizing damage to other workers and patients. temp today 98.2

Journal of the Plague Year, Day 481. A little more learning from history, although I may have told this story before (us old folks repeat ourselves a lot). Years ago all long term care facility staff were asked to get flu shots annually. Many didn't get it. Then the state, which regulates these facilities, said if you don't get the vaccine you have to wear a mask. You can still avoid the shot, but you have to wear a mask for several months during flu season. At my facility, virtually every staff member, except for a few with clearly medical reasons, then took the vaccine. It wasn't a heavy handed imposition or taking away rights, just a rule to improve the safety of residents. Studies showed that if you vaccinate staff with flu shots you got better results than if you vaccinated residents. So when you put a tiny little pressure on those who waver, you get results. Of course, there was nobody years ago who said the flu was a hoax. temp today 98.6

Journal of the Plague Years, Day 482. So, with all the carrots and the sticks I've documented in the last few days, how are things going? Again, I'll use the assisted living where I work as an example. Around January, the vaccines became available. 95% of the residents took it and about 54% of the staff. The staff acceptance was pretty disappointing. But since then, the numbers have changed. The 4-5 residents who didn't take it then are still refusing. But the % of staff who have taken it has gone from 54 to about 86%. this is well above the 70% the city is aiming at. And it's likely to go higher. If a dozen more staff take it, we'll have 100% vaccinated. This was without major carrots or sticks, just people realizing it was the right thing to do. Let's hope this example spreads to the rest of the city and country. temp today 98.3

Journal of the Plague Years, Day 483. Yesterday I went into the subway at 110th and Lenox and saw lots of cops. 3-4 near the turnstile were giving a ticket to a young guy who didn't have a mask. Further down the platform 4 more were giving a ticket to another guy who was wearing one, at least at the time they had him. I'm not sure if the tickets were for mask violations or something else. I briefly felt sorry for the guys getting the tickets, but then I though that if they were acting like jerks and not wearing masks they deserved the tickets. But enforcement of the rules doesn't seem to work too well when at least 4 of the cops had no masks anywhere on their faces at all. It's hard to enforce rules when you don't believe them yourself. And, while writing these tickets, at least three mask less people walked by the cops and they did nothing. As I've said before, and will probably have to say again many times, enforcement of the subway rules is very inconsistent. Maybe they're just looking for violent acts, spot enforcement of various rules here or there, or who knows what. temp today 98.6

Journal of the Plague Years, Day 484. A little more on the "back to normal" theme. Every year we give our residents and staff flu shots. Nurses from the Community Nursing Department, I think, come up from Mount Sinai bringing vaccines with them. Last year, during covid, these nurses and some of our own, went to individual apartments to give the flu shots, and staff got them in our main activity/meeting room. Quarantine is now gone, at least right now, and so we can do it the pre-covid way. One day, probably in November, all the residents and staff will come to the activity room and there will be several staff members there on an assembly line set up. First, everyone signs permission, answers questions (have a fever, allergic to eggs?, etc) and waits for one of the several nurses to give them the shot. I've always thought this communal set up was very good for moral, since it demonstrates that all of us are together when it comes to prevention. I wait for the place to get crowded and that's when I go and get my shot so that patients and staff can see that I practice what I preach and my nagging them is not just words. I also depend on the yentas in the room to spread the word that I was there also, and so get maximum communication to the whole facility. I just hope that delta spread doesn't put us back into quarantine before this happens. temp today 98.4

Journal of the Plague Years, Day 487, Monday August 2. I've tried to think up something original to post but right now there's only one story. The delta strain is making things worse everywhere and what steps to stop or slow it. City and State are mandating vaccines or employees will have to take weekly covid tests. This isn't a big problem, we did it at our ALF, but it's a nuisance so maybe people will give in and get the vaccine. The vaccine isn't that difficult either with minimal side effects, at least when compared to almost any other medication you can take. The City won't hire new people unless vaccinated. More mask wearing indoors, although not mandated. There are endless permutations of these restrictions, trying to not piss people off while trying to keep people alive. I'll try to give all the bad news at the start of the week and the good news by Friday. I hope there is some good news by Friday. temp today 98.3

Journal of the Plague Years, Day 488. Not that much is happening at my facility, but lots of things are happening everyplace else. The city is starting to bring in some type of mandate that masks should be worn when indoors. Some health clubs and restaurants are refusing to admit anyone who is not vaccinated. Some city and state agencies are requiring unvaccinated staff to get weekly covid tests. All these steps will help. Vaccines and NPIs (non-pharmacological interventions) are the tools we have. They are as effective as anything you will see in any aspect of medicine. If people don't use them (and I don't just mean people in Florida) things will get worse, and if people start to use them more things will eventually get better. Few things in medicine are this simple. temp today 98.1

Journal of the Plague Years, Day 489. I've posted a lot about NYC coming back, and last night I decided to look for some other people's takes on this issue. If you have Spectrum as your cable TV provider then you should get CUNY TV channel 75. At 10-11 on weekday nights there is a show called the Stoler Report. It's a bunch of real estate developers talking about trends in real estate around NYC. Last night Stoler, the host, had three developers talking about retail businesses after covid. It was a rerun from the end of March but their attitude was very upbeat. 2008 had a wide spread economic collapse that effected lots of people, but this pandemic still allowed for a lot of people working at home and keeping their incomes flowing. They felt that all this cash that couldn't be spent during quarantine would now be available to spark a resurgence in the local economy. This would help everything from small mom and pop stores to fancy places and even some larger ones (Whole Foods, Trader Joes, etc). They didn't foresee the closing of Kmart recently, but then again since it was immediately replaced by Wegman's their prediction seemed reasonable. This, of course, would only effect those places that weathered the year and a half (or more?)

that it would take for the pandemic to completely end. I'm going to keep watching and see what they say about residential housing bounce back. temp today 98.7

Journal of the Plague Years, Day 490. Nazis! Freedom! You'll get my vaccination card when you pry it from my cold dead hands! NYC is soon going to require people going indoors for restaurants or bars to be vaccinated or be banned and people act like it's some unprecedented infringement on freedom. We all got carded to make sure we were of legal drinking age when we were young. Nobody screamed "Nazis" at the guys working the doors. Many of us got patted down and searched for weapons when we went into clubs years ago. Nobody thought it was an infringement on our constitutional rights. In fact, I always was reassured when I was patted down because that meant that all the other mooks going into the place were also patted down and were weapon free. With delta spreading around and killing people, these minor precautions, no worse than those we have endured forever, will save lives. Not "may" save lives, they will save lives. Get vaccinated and carry your vaccine proof with you like you carry your drivers license, car registration, and picture ID. Or, avoid these precautions and help to kill people. temp today 98.3

Journal of the Plague Years, Day 491. I try to end the week on an upbeat note, but this week has been difficult. The only significant silver lining in this bleak dark cloud has been that the same states that have big increases in covid are also having big increases in vaccinations. It would have been better to do this before the cases increased but better late than never. And by never, I mean after you're dead when a vaccine won't help you. This is also in spite of bad behavior and misinformation from idiot governors and certain media outlets. I hope that this current phase of the race between the virus and vaccinations resolves quickly before the next mutant, lamda I think it's called, hits us. temp today 98.7

Journal of the Plague Years, Day 494, Monday August 9th. After dinner yesterday I took a yellow cab (the only type I usually use) to get home. The driver was friendly and talkative and when I asked my usual question..."how's business" he gave me an earful. He said that at one time there were 18,000 yellow cab drivers, and now only 5000. My own internet search gave a drop of 12,000 to 3,000 but that was only for the covid period and not the Uber/Lyft damage done previously. Like before, customers in the theater district and midtown were rare, but down town areas with lots of bars and restaurants were busier. Before covid, leasing a taxi from the fleet owners cost $6-800 for an 8 hour shift. Now they are leasing for $350-400 for a 24 hour shift. Fleet owners had the advantage before, but now with lack of customers and lack of drivers, those who are still driving have the advantage. He said that with a big smile. temp today 98.2

Journal of the Plague Years, Day 495. The talkative taxi driver went on. One of the reasons, he said, that drivers were willing to take out million dollar loans to get medallions was partially due to speculation. Fleet owners had bought medallions years ago when they were cheaper and when the market price hit one million some cashed out and made a killing just on this speculation. Drivers may have thought they could do the same and hold on to the medallions as they went up and up to 2 million, while using them to make a living. But, the market value leveled off and only a handful of people picked up on it and realized it was about to crash. Then Uber and Lyft came in, accelerating the crash, then covid came in and put the final nail in the yellow taxi's coffin. But, it's not over yet since Revel is bringing in 500 cars to add to the mix, although I'm not sure how they will be used. Trying to make a killing in a bubble is not new. People do it in the stock market all the time, the real estate market, and someone as smart as Sir Isaac Newton got burned in the Dutch Tulip craze centuries ago. The driver said he wasn't taken in, and only leased his taxi, never buying it. He said this with a big smile also. temp today 98.7

Journal of the Plague Year, Day 496. I wonder about life after the plague. I've posted about the economy recovering and people moving back into the city (meaning Manhattan). There are smaller changes that have been made during quarantine that I really wish will disappear when we try to get back to normal. One is subway token booths taking cash again and helping us with expired or partially filled Metrocards. This is minor for me, as I have a Seniors card, but for others it's a real pain. Another is museums requiring reservations to get visit. I don't like having to make reservations to get into a museum and I really hate having to do it on line. When the weather was nice I would sometimes leave work early (it's good to be the doctor-a recurring theme) and walk from my office on 108th street and Fifth avenue back to my apartment at the end of Perry Street. About 5 miles. I could do it casually since I have membership in many museums and I could go from the Guggenheim to the Met to Whitney (before they moved) to MOMA and then home. I could go at my own pace and linger as long as I wanted where ever I wanted. With reservations I'll have my eye on the clock at a time that I want to be relaxed and informal. OK, this is a relatively minor inconvenience during a plague where people are dying by the millions, but it's a minor inconvenience that should be easy to correct. At least I hope so. I miss those walks down Fifth Avenue. temp today 98.5

Journal of the Plague Year, Day 498. Good news Friday! I was speaking to the manager of the dining room at our facility. During quarantine meals were brought to rooms three times a day. People were isolated and many weren't eating much. Now the dining room is open again to everyone. Well, almost. The three residents who refused the vaccine are usually put on a separate table, but everyone else can come and mingle. Each meal has a two hour window and they can come any time except the last 15 minutes if possible, as the staff has to clean up. They can sit where they want with whoever they want. The result is that they are almost all showing up, even the habitual hermits. They are eating everything, even the previously really picky eaters are now cleaning their plates. The social setting, the resumption of freedom, and the beautiful view overlooking Central Park are producing unexpected good results. Residents have taken to the new situation like crazy. Eventually there may be social spats about who sits with who or they will get bored with the food or whatever (like the dining rooms some of us sat in during middle or high school) but right now we're getting good results. Hope it lasts. temp today 98.4

Journal of the Plague Year, Day 501, Monday August 16. To follow up the last post about our dining room. I was glad that it reopened and people are enjoying it. But it illustrates a new way of looking at our post-covid future. I have been thinking about how we could get back to the pre-covid normal. But I haven't been conscious of the fact that things might actually be better than before. For example, when old people lose their appetites either due to illness, depression, or the medications we give them, it's sometimes very hard to get them to resume eating. We loosen dietary restrictions, start to get them supplements (Ensure, Boost, etc), bring in their favorites foods, and lots of other tricks. Sometimes even medications (Megace, THC, yes, THC) usually with poor results. But the dining room results show that sometimes something as simple as socialization is enough. So many of our residents have been partially or completely socially isolated during the quarantine that the opportunity to meet with others is discovered to be more enjoyable than it has ever been before. Socialization was taken for granted, and so undervalued. Now it is rediscovered and people, even a few of our previously hermit behaving residents, are appreciating it a lot more. I hope this continues. temp today 97.6

Journal of the Plague Years, Day 502. A few months ago I posted about going to Macy's main store and how depressing it was to see it so empty. Last Friday, the 13th I went back to buy some stuff and this is what I found. The main floor had a decent amount of customers walking around, although I'm not exact sure how this would compare to pre-covid crowds. Up on the floors it was different. One floor had only a few customers and few sales people, although it had a stock of the item I wanted. On another floor there was only floor samples with no supplies in stock, and there were no bags at the register. It seemed that they were simply not ready for prime time. So, it was mixed. Some improvement on the main floor and pretty empty on the other floors. I'll go back again, but I'm not sure when. It both cases, the choices I had for the items I wanted wasn't anywhere near what is available on their wed site. Macy's is fighting Amazon by becoming Amazon, at least a little bit. temp today 98.5

Journal of the Plague Years, Day 503. On the news tonight a story of two parents who left their kid in the back seat of a car while they went shopping. The kid didn't die, but they were still arrested, probably for criminal negligence, reckless endangerment, endangering the welfare of a child or whatever. They may even lose custody of the kid. You now have governors who are putting their entire states into the back seat of a car, engaging in criminal acts similar to those parents. But the difference is that in these states people actually are dying. Texas and Florida account for 40% of new covid cases while being about 15% of the US population. I wish these governors would end up in jail, or at the very least lose custody of their states. I've tried to stick to only medical opinion in these posts and avoid toxic politics even when it is called for. But, it's getting harder to do. Along with lack of vaccination and immunosupression, having a R********* governor seems to be a major risk factor for covid infection and death. Sad. temp today 98.6

Journal of the Plague Year, Day 504. Lots of developments in fighting covid. We're using carrots and sticks, tools to make it easier to fight and voluntary (carrots) and tools which require actions (sticks). tonight, sticks. By September all healthcare workers in nursing homes, assisted living facilities and other healthcare settings will be required to get vaccines. No longer voluntary. Facilities which don't comply will lose Medicare and

Medicaid payments which will be a death sentence for virtually all nursing homes. It's essentially an unavoidable mandate. In NYC everyone who go into restaurants, gyms and entertainment venues, will have to show proof of vaccinations. By September enforcement will start, which I assume means health department or liquor authority inspectors will inspect sites and maybe pull their licenses if there isn't compliance. That's what happened to the White Horse Tavern, briefly, and what happened at Gem Spa candy store before it closed. A few places lose their licenses and you will see immediate compliance by almost everyone else. Maybe. Tomorrow, carrots to make covid control easier. temp today 97.6

Journal of the Plague Years, Day 505. So, what is making it easier to fight covid? The biggest voluntary option, consistent with the "carrot" metaphor, is the upcoming availability of a third shot, a booster. Annual boosters for flu, and other boosters for tetanus, pneumonia and other diseases are widely used in medicine so this isn't some unprecedented development. At my ALF we are ready to give the third shot to about six people who are severely immune suppressed and by the start of October we should be able to give it to all of our residents because they are all over 65. When we gave the first two shots about 95% of the residents took them, and we probably will get a similar number with this. Also, eventually, we may be able to give the third shot to the staff also, but guidelines on that haven't been announced yet. By the way, some results are in concerning the first round of shots. This week, covid testing was done on about one half of the residents at our facility who voluntarily asked for it. Every one was negative for covid. In spite of the loosening guidelines for quarantine, staff and visitors (all potential carriers) going in and out, and residents going in and out for various reasons, we were 100% negative for this population. The half of residents who didn't get the voluntary test might have a case here or there, but we haven't seen any cases yet. Good news. This stuff works, usually. temp today 97.7

Journal of the Plague Year, Day 508, Monday August 23rd. Both the carrot and the stick have advanced today and I've had trouble keeping up with all of them. The Pfizer vaccine has gotten final approval so maybe those people who were waiting for this will now get vaccinated. Or maybe not. More mandatory vaccinations ("you must...") for the military, NYC teachers, nursing home and hospital employees, etc are being announced every day and it's hard to keep up with the details for each one. Other semi-mandatory vaccinations ("you must, or you will have to do this...") like New Jersey school personnel having to get the vaccines or have masking and weekly testing, are being instituted also. Weekly testing and consisted mask wearing is a pain but not impossible, since we did it at my ALF job site and it may have contributed to very good results documented on previous posts many months ago. More ease of vaccine arrangements and more mandatory rules are going to come out and it will be hard to track them. I'll try to concentrate on what the DOH is requiring for my facility, since that's what I'll know best. temp today 98.1

Journal of the Plague Years, Day 509. Yesterday I posted about national trends, today just what's going on in the ALF where I work. We are starting to see respiratory infections in some of our patients and have to decide if we handle them like we did before covid, or go the whole covid protocol route. The DOH does not allow us to test them, either with the fast 15 minute test or the pcr test that takes a few days. Monoclonal antibodies have been described as something that can be given to prevent hospitalizations, but the DOH has given us no guidelines on this and our pharmacy does not have the antibody in stock for routine use. So, when somebody comes down with respiratory symptoms, we have to decide to treat them at the ALF or send them to the ER. Here, the DOH has given guidelines with minor symptoms, major symptoms, or critical symptoms all triggering different levels of response ranging from treat in place up to ER transfer. I don't know how this will actually work since some of these symptoms are not so clear cut but as we go into fall and winter we will soon find out how useful they are. I just hope that covid dies down enough so that if we misjudge an individual case we don't end up killing someone. temp today 97.9

Journal of the Plague Year, Day 510. "The presence of the hangman's noose focuses the mind considerably" paraphrase of quotation by Samuel Johnson. The same is true of the presence of illness. Today, six high risk patients and myself got the third dose of the Pfizer vaccine. In a few weeks 95% of the remaining patients will receive the third dose. They all voluntarily agreed to the third dose. 95% is a much higher acceptance rate than nursing home and hospital staff, the military, police and fire fighters, or the general US population (not to mention the residents of Texas or Florida). Even those with dementia and their families, understood the seriousness of covid and no conspiracy theory, vaccine fear, anti-v** philosophy, or political motivation was going to dissuade them. They are old and know illness and death, and the presence of morbidity and mortality focused their minds considerably. I wish the rest of the country would come to the same realization. temp today 98.0

Journal of the Plague Year, Day 511. (A little late) I've been waiting to write this while I gather more direct information. It appears to me that there are fewer cops in the subways. A few weeks ago, or maybe a month or two, there were usually many cops on several stations during my rush hour trips. Last week on one day I saw four cops. Today I saw another four. But, this is a lot less than previously. I haven't read anything in the papers about a decrease in subway policing, but I'm only going by what I see during my trips. Maybe they are somewhere else, or on the trains or other parts of the stations, but I don't know where they would be that I wouldn't see them. I'll keep my eyes open but remember, if the papers announce that police have been taken out of the subways you heard it here first. temp today 98.9

Journal of the Plague Years, Day 512. It's hard to make this Friday's post upbeat, but I can at least make it light instead of somber. SNL used to have a recurring skit called "White People's Problems" where some "problem" would be discussed by a bunch of white folks that was so trivial that the black cast members would break out laughing. Here's a few covid related ones. First, remote delivery. Food delivered to my apartment and my newspapers in the morning have to be left in the lobby and I have to come down and get them. I'm on the second floor, so it's not a big trip. A very trivial inconvenience. Second, restaurants whose menus have to be accessed by QR codes read by your cell phone instead of paper menus. Also trivial, although I have seen people leave restaurants when they were required to use QR instead of paper. Third, having to wear masks at multiple locations (subways, indoor meetings, gyms, etc). A little more inconvenient but pretty easy when you get used to it. Fourth, making reservations to be able to walk into a museum. Many of these are slowly being loosened up and may or may not disappear after covid. But they are mostly minor when compared to the morbidity and mortality of covid. So minor, in fact, that they could easily be classified as "White People's Problems" metaphorically if not literally. temp today 97.9

Journal of the Plague Years, Day 515, Monday August 30. Last week the city began requiring restaurants to ask for vaccination proof when entering for indoor dining. I went to three of my favorite places to test this out: Piccolo Angolo on Hudson street, Cafe Katja on Orchard, Cafe Palermo on Mulberry. All three were asking for proof. Since I was eating and drinking I may not have been able to verify that every single person was carded, but it seemed that most people were pulling out their vaccine cards or showing something on their cell phones, where there are apps for vaccine proofs. It seems these three places were trying their best to comply. I don't know if this effected their business since August is always a very slow month in NYC. I was glad to show off my vaccine card with three lines filled in (two for the initial vaccination and the third for the recent booster I got). Not every business is so compliant and I'll look at them tomorrow. temp today 97.9

Journal of the Plague Years, Day 516. I was ready to post about bad behavior related to vaccine carding for restaurants but The Village Sun, an on-line news source for the West Village beat me to it. Patiscerria Rocco has a branch in Brooklyn and one in the West Village, the last Italian pastry shop in the Village. The owner is proclaiming that she will not require vaccination proof for inside eating. She says this is not political but she is standing up for freedom, although she said it at a rally attended by Curtis Sliwa the R********* candidate for mayor. The sign outside her Village branch says she won't discriminate against anyone on the basis or race or sex or whether they are vaccinated. She forgot to mention that she also is not discriminating against selfish individuals who are willing to give other people an infectious disease that might kill them. How nice of her. To verify this public announcement, I went into the Village branch and offered my vaccine card to the waiter but he waved it off not even willing to look at it. I'll miss their cannolis and panettones, but I won't be going back there again until after covid, or maybe not ever depending how pissed off I am when this is over. It's behavior by shop owners like her that are prolonging this epidemic for everyone and killing a lot of people that could have been saved by prevention. temp today 97.9

Journal of the Plague Years, Day 517. The conflict between pro-v***** restaurants and anti-v***** places might be decided in September when enforcement is supposed to start. I haven't been able to find out exactly how enforcement will work. Will health inspectors, which the city has plenty of, set up sting operations to catch people breaking the rules, as they did to Gem Spa and lead to them losing their cigarette license for a while? Will they downgrade the letter rankings of places? Lots of places like to show off their A ratings, but what happens if that goes down to B or C or D, if there even is a D? Will they get fined? Will they get multiple fines? Can the DOH close a business as a health hazzard? Will they pull liquor licenses like they did to the White Horse Tavern, which scared the shit out of the other restaurants on Hudson street? Or will they just shrug because their are too many violators and enforcement is too much of a pain. To paraphrase the end of the movie Chinatown: "Forget it Jake, it's covid." We'll see. temp today 98.4

Journal of the Plague Years, Day 518. The restaurant owners who are anti-v*******, or who won't enforce vaccine documentation, might learn a little from history. In 2013 a restaurant in The Bronx, New Hawaii Sea (previously South Sea restaurant) on Williamsbridge road had a worker who was infected with hepatitis A. Due to poor sanitation at the restaurant, it spread to a few other workers and customers. When it became public, everyone who worked or ate food from the place were encouraged to get hepatitis A vaccinations or gamma globulin injections. Hundreds, and possibly thousands, got the shots. Some people got sick and sued the restaurant. It went out of business and was eventually replaced by a sushi restaurant. This all started with ONE employee. And covid is much more lethal than hepatitis A. If a restaurant is sloppy with the vaccination rules and just ONE worker or customer spreads covid to others it could end up killing someone and destroying the business also. Anti-v****** act as if these rules have no purpose except to make life difficult for them. They're wrong. temp today 98.0

Journal of the Plague Years, Day 519. I don't know if this will be a positive ending to the week but it is a significant development, at least for me. Recently, the DOH required all hospital and nursing home staff to get vaccinated, but assisted living and senior housing staff were excluded from that mandate. No more. A recent DOH decision requires all ALF staff to be vaccinated by early October or be fired. The ALF where I work has started to work with the staff to make sure they get their shots, but those who don't have it by October will be fired. Also, they will be fired for cause which means they probably won't be able to get unemployment insurance. This seems extreme and imposes a burden on employees. But, there are other milder impositions on staff to get their annual flu vaccines and get tested for TB annually and there is 100% compliance with those rules. Getting the vaccine for covid is easy with virtually no risk of significant side effects, but being susceptible to having or spreading covid is potentially deadly. And by "deadly" I don't mean it as a metaphor, I mean it literally. To neutralize the amount of misinformation by anti-v****** a gentle suggestion is no longer enough. Now there has to be enforcement . temp today 97.9

Journal of the Plague Year, Day 523, Tuesday September 7. Let's start with potentially bad news. It will be better by Friday. The DOH of NY sends out letters to doctors on a variety of topics from mosquito spraying to covid rules. Last week I got a letter saying that doctors caring for refugees from Afghanistan should watch out for cases of measles and polio. Polio! I don't know how much of these exist in Afghanistan but I know there is polio in Pakistan, right next door. The last polio case originating in the US was 1979 and the last time a case was brought into the US by a traveler was 1993. So no polio in almost 30-40 years. When a measles outbreak happened in Disneyland a few years back, lots of anti-v****** went out and finally got vaccines. If a single case of polio were to pop up in the US, by refugees or just visitors from Pakistan or Nigeria, the whole v***** vs anti-v***** debate would become much more significant. Having one preventable epidemic going around the country is bad enough, but to have one or two more preventable outbreaks would be so much worse. temp today. 98.5

Journal of the Plague Year, Day 524. Around the corner from my apartment in the normally liberal West Village there was a parked Volvo with big decal letters that spelled out "Don't Fauci My Child." It had NY plates, so it wasn't a visitor from Texas or Florida, but presumably a local resident. This is so sad. Since this slogan is pretty vague I don't know if they are referring to mask wearing, social distancing, or vaccines. If it's vaccines then these parents should lose custody of their kids. Harsh? If a parent ignored safety precautions and left a child in the back seat of a car in the hot sun that parent could be charged with child abuse, reckless endangerment or criminal negligence. If the kid died, the parents could be charged with manslaughter on the basis of these same crimes. I hope that when the vaccine becomes available for kids under 12, these parents would be sane enough to get the kid vaccinated. If not, maybe the kids school would require it. I would hate to see the epitaph "We Didn't Fauci Our Child" on the kids gravestone. temp today 98.1

Journal of the Plague Year, Day 525. Yesterdays post about the "Don't Fauci My Child" made me realize that those of us who are sane and don't want to kill people need a similar simple motto. How about "WhatWouldFauciDo?" or just "WWFD?". Fauci isn't perfect and has, and will, make mistakes. But a motto (or would this be considered a meme if there is no picture?) or slogan isn't supposed to be a detailed logical dissection, but a tool to present a simple clear idea. Listen to people who have been doing this work mostly correctly for 50 years. Listen to science. Listen to objectivity. I don't know how to spread this motto. I put it on Twitter as #whatwouldfaucido? and #wwfd? but I don't know how to spread it (make it "viral" if you pardon the metaphor). So Facers reading this and Twitterers who are on that platform, please help this computer impaired person spread this. temp today 99.1

Journal of the Plague Year, Day 526. There were various uplifting things I could post about, but one happened right after I had dinner and was walking home. At about 7:30 I passed Hudson street between Perry and Charles and in the street, next to the outdoor dining sheds, was a four piece brass band playing some lively music (I don't even remember what because of the red wine at the dinner I just finished). They were entertaining the packed sidewalk and shed tables filled with dinners. I dropped a buck in their bucket and walked home. I don't know if this sidewalk busking started in NYC with the outdoor covid dining, but it seems to have given it a little boost. Any Facers around my neighborhood, or anywhere else, who sees these folks and others like them, drop a buck. They're not beggers, just plain entertainers and might actually make the city a more pleasant place. temp today 98.2

Journal of the Plague Years, Day 529, Monday Sept 13th. Usually, I enjoy scooping the media to some piece of news. Not this time. On Sept 7 I posted about a warning from the NY DOH about Afghan refugeees possibly having measles or polio and how health care providers should be on the watch for these possibilities. This Saturday, the 11th, the Times had an article about four Afhan refugees who had active cases of measles and were put into querantine will tracing was done to see if they had infected anyone. Measles sounds benign, but it can kill. I wish I had been wrong and the alarms were simply over caution, but it looks like the problem wasn't just theoretical. And this is nothing compared to what will happen if a case of polio gets into the US. temp today 97.1

Journal of the Plague Year, Day 530. The NHY DOH had a webinar recently for providers concerning data on covid. There was a lot included so I'll take it one topic at a time. First, delta variant and vaccines. 98% of covid in NYC is delta. The vaccine, however, protects against covid. As a result, the areas with the lowest vaccine rates (southern Staten Island, City Island, west Rockaways) have the high rates of covid and the highest rates of hospitalizations. They didn't break it down by deaths, but hospitalizations might be a very rough measure of deaths. Complete vaccinations are not 100% effective and there are occasionally deaths in vaccinated individuals. This NYC data said unvaccinated have ten times the death rate of vaccinated but other data around the country show the ratio of unvax/vax even higher than 10 to one. I'll have to keep looking for more detailed data. The bottom line? Get vaccinated. Not a very original idea, but true none the less. temp today 97.7

Journal of the Plague Years, Day 531. More on the covid webinar. Monoclonal antibodies, abbreviated mAB, to covid are available and being increasingly used. They are designed to be used before a patient goes to the hospital to prevent the hospitalization and death. If you have a positive covid test, getting mAB will decrease hospitalizations and death by 70-85% depending on what survey you see. If people are exposed to an active case and have no symptoms overall cases are reduced by 66-81% (I'm not sure about deaths). If symptoms or exposure persist, this can be given (by IV or sub-cutaneous injection) every four weeks. If the person previously had covid or had the complete vaccine, it can still be given for new break through cases. When used correctly this treatment looks pretty effective, even if not 100% effective. It's so good even T**** took it! temp today 98.7

Journal of the Plague Years, Day 532. This post will seem very trivial, but I've been looking forward to it for a while. As the city has slowly been coming back to normal, I have been using the behavior on the subway as an indirect measurement of recovery. I've looked at the Times Square subway station, on the 2 and 3 lines, and noticed how empty the station was. We would pull into the station and by the time we left we would be more empty than when we entered. I took this to mean that midtown was empty. No theater crowd, tourists, or office workers. Today, for the first time that I noticed, the train left with more passengers from 42nd street that it had before. Pulling into the station, with every seat taken (although there were seats empty on both sides of every sitter) there were 13 standees. Pulling out, there were 18. OK, this isn't the most scientific study, but it was the first time I noticed this change. Three people with luggage going to Penn station, one mother with two kids, and a bunch of people whose background I couldn't judge. Is this a trend? One day means little, but I hope it does predict the future. I'll keep watching, and counting. temp today 98.3

Journal of the Plague Years, Day 533. Along with my posts, you may have been reading those of Trigger Thompson, a Burner who is opening up ice cream storefronts in the middle of this epidemic around lower Manhattan. He recently opened his second one on St. Mark's Place in the East Village, to join the one already opened on Delancey street, and to be joined by another one on Division street in the future. It doesn't take much to see that the fate of three little ice cream places doesn't amount to a hill of beans in this crazy world (yes, that's a paraphrase of Rick's speech to Ilsa in the final scene of Casablance. Plenty of useful quotes from that movie.) But it goes along with a theme I've been using since the start of this pandemic, that of resilience of NYC. Good luck to Trigger and the countless other small businesses that are opening up all over the city right now. I would be shocked, shocked, if many of them didn't succeed. temp today 98.7

Journal of the Plague Years, Day 536, Monday Sept 20. Last week the San Gennaro feast returned to Little Italy in NYC. It had been closed last year due to covid, but organizers thought this year would be safe. I was there last week a few times. It was crowded but I couldn't tell if it was because there were more people or the streets were narrow due to side walk dining. John Fratta who helps organize the feast said the crowds were actually bigger. This years feast was dedicated to the first responders of NYC along with San Gennaro himself. During my visits there I ate too much sausage, bracciole, calzone, and pastry, which is typical. I'm so weak when it comes to food. It was good to see this 95 year old tradition back, and it will last until Sunday Sept 26. But, was it dangerous? Tune in tomorrow. temp today 97.9

Journal of the Plague Year, Day 537. So, is the San Gennaro feast dangerous? Let's take the bad news first. On three visits to the feast it was always packed. People were side by side breathing near each other. It was outdoors but still people were still breathing on each other, and presumably coughing on each other now and then. This reminded me of the motorcycle rally in Sturgis where a similar crowd was squeezed together. In the feast less than 5% of the crowd or the vendors staffing the booths were masked, according to my unscientific observation. In the whole feast I only saw one cop with a mask, every other one was without a mask. The indoor restaurants lined Mulberry street's entire length and I'm note sure if every single one was asking for vaccine proof like they were supposed to do. There could have been pockets of spreaders tucked away in one bar or restaurant or another. I hope this doesn't turn out to be a super spreader, like Sturgis, or even a mini-spreader. We'll find out in a few weeks. Tomorrow, I give the good news. temp today 97.5

Journal of the Plague Years, Day 538. Now some good news about San Gennaro and some things that might decrease the chance of it being a super spreader event. The weather has been great and except for tomorrow, Thursday, it will remain so. Covid spreads less when everyone is outdoors instead of inside. Probably a lot of the restaurants are checking vaccine cards, although I can't know how many. Both NYC and New Jersey have vaccination rates of about 70% getting at least one shot, which is a pretty good rate. Also, NYC has an overall covid positive test rate of about 1% which is pretty good also, although there are some reports of it rising recently. In other words, covid spreads the most in areas where it already exists or areas where few people are vaccinated. Neither applies to NYC or the San Gennaro feast. The odds aren't zero for spread via the feast, but they are about as low as you can get for an event like this. I hope I'm right. temp today 98.3

Journal of the Plague Years, Day 539. Two steps forward, one step back. I was looking forward to the annual convention of the Gerontological Society of America convention in Phoenix this November. In person! Well, too good to be true. This week I got an email that said that it would be remote, not in person. I was disappointed, but understanding. Although the covid rate in Arizona is just a little high, it doesn't mean that Phoenix or the confined convention center wouldn't be a potential danger zone. It also wasn't clear what would be the situation in the middle of

November when the convention was supposed to happen. So, all virtual for now. Well, two more conventions next year. The American Medical Directors Association in Baltimore in March and the American Geriatric Society in Orlando in May. Wish me luck. I'm really tired of remote meetings. temp today 96.7

Journal of the Plague Years, Day 540. Good news Friday. Was it the FDA or CDC that approved vaccine booster shots? With deaths approaching 700,000 every addition layer of protection is needed. Right now the approval is for people over 65, like me, and those with special medical conditions. The CDC head added boosters for front line health care workers, also like me. Needless to say, I got my booster already wince we knew this was coming and I'm walking around, and showing off, a vaccine card with three lines filled in. B**** was attacked for saying everyone should get the booster, but he was only ahead of the curve, not wrong. Eventually everyone will get the booster. Medical literature and data presented at some of the virtual meetings I've gone to, show that immunity starts to decrease after 6 months and at some point might become ineffective. It's not like some vaccines or infections that are good for a lifetime. So, get everything you can get as soon as you can get it, and keep doing every precaution (masks!) when possible. Good luck. temp today 99.1 (don't worry, 99.1 is not a real fever).

Journal of the Plague Years, Day 543, Monday Sept 27. I may have posted about this before, a long time ago, but I received some confirmation yesterday. Facers reading this know I talk to my taxi drivers when coming home from dinner at times. Yesterday's driver mentioned that he will be wearing his mask all the time, even after covid is gone. He said he gets 4-5 colds and coughs every winter but this year got none. So, he'll keep safe with his mask as we come into winter and fall. I've also had none of my usual 4-5 coughs/colds/sinus infections this year. My patients haven't had any. My own doctor says he has seen almost none all year. We don't have vaccines for all these viruses, so the only thing accounting for this is the NPIs (non-pharmacological interventions like masks, isolation, etc) are keeping us safe. And all those years I laughed at the Koreans and Japanese who used to mask up every winter. They were right. temp today 97.7

Journal of the Plague Years, Day 544. Yesterday I posted about how precautions can help with covid and many other respiratory diseases. What happens if something goes wrong? Today I learned that one of the staff at the facility where I worked tested positive for covid after feeling a little sick on Friday. Everyone resident of the facility who had been in contact had to go on isolation. That means 17 people have to stay in their rooms, get meds and food delivered, and avoid other people as much as possible. This is being very careful as all of the 17 residents, except one I think, had the vaccine and even if sick were not likely to be very sick. On the other hand, they could have gotten very sick so we had to be careful. This started with one positive case, the staff member. This disease can still spread easily, still make people sick, still kill. We can't let down our guard even in widely vaccinated populations. temp today 98.3

Journal of the Plague Years, Day 545. One more post about our ability to control infectious respiratory diseases. I've posted about how there was a big drop in respiratory diseases (colds, coughs, flu, pneumonia, etc) last winter before the covid vaccine came out. Almost totally gone were my infections, my patients, my doctors patients, staff at the ALF where I work, my taxi driver from last Sunday. One more piece of evidence. The drug store where I go to get my own medications (nothing serious-Crestor and vitamin D) said that last winter there was a tremendous drop in meds for those problems. Less antihistamines, decongestants, cough syrups, antibiotics. Every thing was down. So, what do we do in the upcoming winter? Will we try and get people to wear masks, self-isolate when they have symptoms, social distance, or what? Will they listen to us when there is no deadly epidemic? As my pharmacist said, "All you can do is lead them in the right direction and hope they do it". We'll see. temp today 97.7

Journal of the Plague Year, Day 546. I was going to move on from talk of decreased respiratory disease, but a letter to doctors from the director of NY DOH came in just today. He was talking about the initial decrease in respiratory diseases among kids, which is not my are of medical practice. From 2019 flu cases among children went from about 60,000 to 6,000 and deaths from 9 to zero. Respiratory synsticial virus (RSV) decreased also even though it commonly attacks kids. This is consistent with what I've reported over the last few days. But over the last few months RSV has increased for 2021. In the medical literature there is worry that the very low rate of respiratory diseases of 2020 might lead to an even worse than average season in 2021 to 2022 since there will be less immunity left over from the 2020 year since there were fewer cases. We don't know if this will happen, but infectious disease docs are worried. We'll find out over the next few months. They are also suggesting we get our flu vaccines and covid boosters both simultaneously and as soon as possible. This is consistent with what I my patients to get every approved treatment you can get as soon as you can get it. temp today 97.6

Journal of the Plague Years, Day 547. This almost sounds too good to be true, but it looks like the Halloween parade in The Village will be back this year. It skipped last year because of covid. For this year they needed to raise about $150,000 and they only had about $10K when Jason and Missy Feldman, either out of their own pockets or some fund raising got them the rest. If this is as good as it sounds this tradition will resume this Halloween. For those of you who read my San Gennaro posts you know that an event like this is not entirely risk free. Most people will not be wearing masks and so there is a risk of it becoming a super spreader or even a mini spreader even. So far, there has been no fall out from San Genarro which ended 2 weeks ago. Let's hope our luck holds out for that event and for Halloween. temp today 97.5

Journal of the Plague Years, Day 550, Monday Oct 4. Last Saturday, on my birthday, I went to see my first Broadway play in almost 2 years. It was called Waitress, a little class warfare, a little feminist outrage, a little rom-com. It was pretty good. The whole experience was a lot like the pre-covid Broadway but a few new things. Everyone had to show vaccine proof and picture ID to get in. Everyone was wearing a mask and the ushers were holding up signs saying "Mask Up" to remind us. There was not social distancing as every seat was taken, all sold out. When I left the theater the crowds outside look pretty substantial and I wouldn't have known there was an epidemic if I didn't know it already. One more step back to normalcy. temp today 98.0

Journal of the Plague Years, Day 551. Like Gaul, the Theater district has three parts. There are the actual theaters which I described last night, the tourists, and the office workers. To sort this out I asked one of my usual sources, a taxi driver. Coming back from the theater I asked "How's business?" He said that the theater crowd was coming back but he was worried about some shows closing even after they opened because someone was infected. He was nervous but still driving. The tourists weren't back yet since the hotels were still pretty empty with little taxi business. He didn't mention the office workers who probably take subways anyway. I told him how fast I was able to get a taxi and he said it was because more drivers are coming back to drive as business slowly picks up. He sounded pretty determined, or maybe resigned, to keep working as the city slowly, slowly reopened. temp today 98.0

Journal of the Plague Years, Day 552. A week or two ago the city announced that it was going to start cracking down on mask wearing in the subways. I thought this was a joke since most of the cops in the subways don't were masks or were them incorrectly. The only time I saw four cops all with masks was when two of them were white shirt supervisors. But it is slowly changing. In the last week I think I seen an increase in total cops but also every one has been wearing a mask, almost all of them wearing it correctly. I haven't seen any cops giving out tickets to the many riders without masks just yet. But getting the cops to mask up is the first step. We'll see if they start enforcing the rules and if everyone starts obeying them. temp today 97.5

Journal of the Plague Years, Day 553. While we're dealing with covid, other diseases are proceeding alone their normal route, and have to be dealt with. This week we have been giving flu shots to our residents. Just plain old fashioned yearly flu shots. About 95% of our residents will take the shot. Each year close to 100% of staff take it, with only a few not taking it because of documented medical reasons. This is because workers who don't take the shot, for whatever reasons, have to wear a mask for the several months of flu season. So, the excuses disappear and they take the shots. 100 residents and about 100 staff take it, little if any significant side effects, and they do it every year, including this year. No big problem, it's just done. If this clear and simple precedent were understood by everyone in the country, covid and the diseases that will someday come after covid, would virtually disappear, as would most Zoom meetings. Jesus, just do it. temp today 96.8

Journal of the Plague Years, Day 554. I haven't been able to do any of my usual travelling this year since Burning Man and several medical conventions have been cancelled or converted to virtual events. So, I've decided to take a real vacation, although only for a few days. I'm going up to Cape Cod this weekend. I often do this in the fall, after Labor Day when the tourist crowds leave, but couldn't do this last year when Massachusetts was locked down. I'm told that's it's mostly opened up now, so I'm heading North. Some of the Facers in this group have been posting pictures from the Cape and nearby islands but I've tracked back on others sites and haven't been able to find pictures. If you have any handy send them for us to see. Meanwhile, I'll try to take some pictures up there and maybe my cousins can teach me how to post them. I'll report back next week, but probably not until I return, maybe about Wednesday. A short break from the city, but better than another Zoom meeting. temp today 97.6

Journal of the Plague Years, Day 559, Wednesday Oct 13. I've just gotten over my hangover from the many wild Columbus Day and Indigenous Peoples parties I've gone to over the last few days, so here's an update from beautiful Cape Cod. I was up there for a few days relaxation and to see my cousins. What's happening with covid? All the bars and restaurants had signs for masking and many people were masked when they entered. The masks usually disappeared once the eating/drinking started. Nobody asked for vaccine proof at any of these places. The crowds of people walking in the streets of Provincetown ("P-town" to the locals) were mostly maskless and my cousins said that this was the most crowded they've seen it since before covid. The TV news news said the covid test rate was 3% but an internet search found a 1.7% number. I'm not sure which is accurate, and I know they're both higher than NY's rate of about 1%, but there seems to be enough control that they feel comfortable not asking for vaccine proof. At least that's the most I can figure out from this little data. I'm sure it's more complicated but that's the best I have. Now, if I can only find an excuse for looking at covid data in New Orleans or San Francisco. temp today 97.9

Journal of the Plague Years, Day 560. In my neighborhood there is a pastry shop, Rocco's, who has a big sign in their window saying they do not discriminate against unvaccinated people and welcome everyone, thus breaking the city mandate of asking for vaccine proof. I've written about this in Westview News (westviewnews.org) and how this is a right wing motivated escalation which could endanger the health of patrons, and possibly cause death. My political club, the Village Independent D******** (village*********.org) just endorsed a letter asking them to reconsider and essentially condemning them for their position. The anti v** movement of this country, virtually all coming from the political right, endangers the health of this country and prolongs the epidemic. It's a shame though, I'll miss their cannolis. But I can't patronize a place that endangers the health of customers and community. temp today 97.2

Journal of the Plague Years, Day 561. When I leave my office on 108th street and Fifth Avenue, I walk along the northern border of Central Park to the subway. This week I've seen something there that I don't remember seeing in the last 18 years I've had this job. New the small pond called the Harlem Meer is a boathouse, and next to it a small open area or plaza. The last few weeks at about 4-5 PM I've seen groups of 10-20 people dancing to Latin music in this small open area. The musicians are there live, as far as I can see, and the people are dancing spontaneously. Maybe this weekend is the time I learn how to post videos to FB so we can all join in. Is this a reaction to covid? I don't know, but it's positive enough that I hope it's a reaction to the possible end of covid, at least in NYC. temp today 98.2

Journal of the Plague Years, Day 564, Monday October 18. Some of these posts have been about major life threatening developments in the covid fight. Today it's a lot more trivial. Before covid my morning papers (News and Times) were delivered to my door. During the quarantine they were all left in the lobby and the deliverer wasn't allowed into the rest of the building. Today, for the first time in a year and a half. the papers were at my door again. It's a pretty small development in our return to normal, but these small symbolic acts give a little psychological re-assurance, as least to me, that the slow slow recovery is at least heading in the right direction. That is, unless there's another spike among the un-vaccinated, a new mutant, and who knows what else. For now, let's take what we can get, including the morning papers. temp today 98.5

Journal of the Plague Years, Day 565. When I went up to Cape Cod recently I took some reading. One book was The Decameron of Boccaccio. The Black Death hit Florence in 1348 and as much as 60% of the population died (covid death rate in the US is about 0.2%). Boccaccio was a writer/poet who lived in the city throughout the plague year. I've only started reading its 600 pages, published in 1353, but there's something to be learned already. He sets the story in Florence where ten friends, 7 women and 3 men join together, flee the city, and end up in one of their nearby castles. These are wealthy folks. Besides the ten narrators they have servants also and so this entire entourage leaves the city and holds up in the castle. For ten nights, each of the ten tells a story on some theme or another, resulting in about 100 stories of various lengths. The stories have little relevance to covid or even to the actual death occurring at the same time. What make's it relevant is that the rich leave town fast. Sound familiar? Tomorrow-Journal of the Plague Year. temp today 96.5

Journal of the Plague Years, Day 566. The second book I read, completely, was "A Journal of the Plague Year." by Daniel DeFoe written in 1722 years after the 1664 plague. It killed maybe as many as 100,000 in London alone, about 1/6th of the population. Although it wasn't an eye witness account, like The Decameron, it is generally historically accurate. What's more, it describes the plague from a ground view, the day to day occurrences within the city. It is written as a novel with the main character who is living through the plague describing what's happening. It covers a lot, but I'll give you a few facts which are relevant to our situation. When the plague started it was in a few districts outside the city and with only a few cases. The officials at the time downplayed the seriousness at first. Sound familiar? When it appeared that it was spreading wealthy individuals who could afford to leave the city did so, even the Royal Court left and went to Oxford to ride out the epidemic. Again, sound familiar. Florence, London, New York, and those with money leave fast. Of course some of them were infected, in all these cases, and probably helped to spread the diseases. More details tomorrow. temp today 97.7

Journal of the Plague Years, Day 567. DeFoe's character describes steps taken by the London city government, which didn't flee but stayed in the city, to control the epidemic. One was to kill all the dogs and cats who they thought spread the disease, and put out extra rat poison for the presumed explosion of the rat population. Although they got the vector wrong, they were aware that something was spreading the plague. Anyone who was found to have plague was forced to stay in their homes and the whole family had to stay with them. Sometimes the doors were actually locked or barred to keep people in. The theory was that the family was exposed anyway so forced quarantine would stop spread throughout the city but not hurt anyone who wouldn't be infected anyway. They knew that it could be spread by person to person contact, which it seems some people today don't want to admit.

Watchmen were hired by the city to stay outside these homes 24 hours a day and enforce the lock down. Sometimes people snuck out anyway, sometimes bribed their way out, and sometimes attacked the watchmen resulting in several deaths. So, the quarantine we had for this epidemic was pretty mild by comparison. Lots of other details were described. As the epidemic subsided, it may have finally been completely ended by the Great London Fire of 1666. Maybe I'll get to Camus' The Plague if I ever finish The Decameron. temp today 97.7

Journal of the Plague Years, Day 568. This Friday's upbeat news is more accurately described as interesting or surprising news. I was walking through Penn station a few days ago in the late afternoon when I heard an overhead announcement (which was actually understandable!) that said that anyone who got the vaccine right then and there would get a one week unlimited Metrocard. For some reason this cheered me up that there were still new ways of encouraging people to get their vaccine shots. I don't know how many took this opportunity, but at least it was there. And this was before the city reportedly offered unvaccinated workers $500 to get the shot. The good news is that the city has not given up on getting people vaccinated, but the bad news is that it's still needed. So today's message is mixed. temp today 97.8

Journal of the Plague Years, Day 571, Monday October 25. This Sunday I saw a large group of people around the corner of Christopher and Bleecker. There is a store on that corner called Whalebone which has a trendy magazine and equally trendy clothing, whisky and ice cream, along with a fascination with Wes Anderson and his movies, such as the recently released "The French Dispatch." The people were lined up for some type of event in the store, at sidewalk tables and under a new awning which said "Le Sans Blague" (No Joke?). I think they even had gift boxes from the event. If I weren't on my way to my morning bagel and if the crowd wasn't so big, I would have investigated. This is another indication that the city, or at least this downtown area, is coming back and is very very busy. That's downtown. What's happening uptown? Tomorrow for that. temp today 97.7

Journal of the Plague Year, Day 572. Yesterday I posted about the lively downtown scene. Uptown, not so much. On the corner of 110th street and Lenox avenue is the Parkview hotel which is used for homeless people. Before covid, I would sometimes see a few people hanging out in front. The last few weeks I've seen 10-20 people there at 9 AM, reading some type of leaflet and looking like they were waiting to go in or to apply. On 109th street off Fifth avenue is the HQ of Common Pantry which dispenses food for needy individuals. Before covid a dozen or so individuals would line up for dispensed food. Now there is often a line of 40-50 that snakes down the block. In both cases the people are all minorities, Black, Hispanic, and Asian. I don't know if this is because of covid but I know it's different than before. Why? Maybe after quarantine, shut down of other services (food banks, SNAP offices, welfare offices, eviction moratoriums, etc) people needing help have just built up their numbers but had nowhere to go. When things opened up, they came out and started lining up for the deferred help they needed. Or maybe it's just a coincidence or I never noticed these people before. I'm trying to describe what I've seen but I don't know exactly how to explain it. I do know one thing. The revival of NYC is not evenly distributed and downtown and uptown are not the same. temp today 98.0

Journal of the Plague Year, Day 573. Last week when I was passing by St. Vincent's/Aids Memorial park on 7th Ave and 12th street, there were some young people there giving out free masks. They were from some city program, although I don't remember the name offhand. They were politely going up to anyone walking by without a mask and offering them cloth masks for free. I've heard there is a similar program in the subways although I haven't seen it myself. Although you don't need a mask outdoors, many stores, restaurants, and bars request that all customers wear a mask when possible. Usually people comply, at least when they first go in before eating and drinking starts. Vaccines did not make masks obsolete or useless, it just pushed them back to second line protection instead of first line protection. But remember, before vaccines NPIs (non-pharmacological interventions) did work so let's not forget them. temp today 97.0

Journal of the Plague Years, Day 574. After the Black Death, so many people died that there was a severe labor shortage and it was given credit for ending the Feudal Period and helping to start the Renaissance. On a smaller level, it is happening again. There are constant reports of labor shortages as workers don't put up with low salaries and bad conditions and are resigning in mass. Many who don't resign are now striking in increasing numbers. this has his long term care like nursing homes and ALFs which have always had a hard time recruiting workers for the same reasons. Today, after the resignation of another aide, I found out that turnover at our place has increased greatly since covid started and we have a hard time replacing workers. Subsidies from Medicaid keep us afloat, but they are low and have gotten lower over the years (thanks Gov. C****!). So, what happens? Hope is that maybe after covid the labor market will stabilize or that with a new governor Medicaid funding will increase. We'll see. Meanwhile, if you know somebody who needs a job like this, get in touch. temp today 97.3

Journal of the Plague Year, Day 575. This week a friend of mine invited me to a fundraising gala for Lifeforce in Later Years (LiLY) which is a non=profit volunteer organization on the Upper West Side that recruits volunteers to help elderly people in the neighborhood in various ways (bringing food, taking to appointments, companionship, etc). The gala though was in person . Not Zoom, internet, remote or anything like that. Actual tables where people sat, ate, drank (open bar), and talked to each other. Everyone was carded for vaccinations, everyone wore masks, at least until the eating/drinking started. I knew a few of the honorees (Dr. Nancy Wexler, Brian Benepe) and a few electeds quietly showed up (Deborah Glick and Gale Brewer). But what a pleasure to be in person. Because of masking/ vaccine precautions the risk of it become a spreader event is really low. Let's hope that's the way it turns our. If so, maybe we can start doing things in person again without going the way of Florida or Texas. Let's hope so. temp today 98.8

Journal of the Plague Years, Day 578, Monday November 1. Yesterday marked the return of the Village Halloween parade. It started at 7 in SoHo but didn't reach Houston and 6th avenue, where I was, until 7:30. The crowds of onlookers were big, at least as big as previous years. Maybe this was due to quarantine exhaustion or just the perfect weather. About 10% of the crowd had masks, and roughly the same % among the cops. The end of the parade passed my viewing spot at 9:30. Some previous parades lasted until 10 or later, but this was a decent showing considering the parade wasn't even sure to go off a few weeks ago. As with other things, if you didn't know about the pandemic this would seem like a typical Halloween parade. Start looking around other pages for the videos that can describe it better than I can. Tomorrow, the high points. temp today 97.9

Journal of the Plague Years, Day 579. The entire Halloween parade is on YouTube, but here are a few highlights from my point of view. The first was Kostume Kults float. Very enthusiastic, wonderful costumes, and this was the group I camped with a few years ago at Burning Man. Many bands from small 6 piece groups to large samba drum bands, brass bands and the Lesbian and large Gay Big Apple Corps who for some reason were wearing lunberjack type jackets and shirts instead of their usual white uniforms. The Thriller dance group was there. About 75 zombies shuffling alone following a sound truck playing Michael Jackson's Thriller. Then the music stops and they all start dancing in perfect unison. Very professional and very impressive. Finally, there was a small religious group with signs saying Worship God, Fear Got not the Virus and various other religious messages. I don't think they meant it sarcastically but were a real fundamentalist organization. That's what I most remember seeing. Tomorrow-what I didn't see at the parade. temp today. 97.7

Journal of the Plague Years, Day 580. What was NOT in the parade? Sometimes the parade can have costumes in very bad taste and very dark. I wondered if there would be anyone dressed up like a covid virus and, thankfully, there wasn't. I didn't see one fake covid virus. Great! But also there was very political content just two days before an election. Our former president appeared twice, once in a jail costume, and our current president not at all. There was one Dr. Fauci that I saw and maybe a few others with big fake hypodermic needles. I'm not sure why this absence since previous parades often had a lot more. Maybe if the parade ran last year a few days before the presidential election there would be more politician costumes since feelings were so intense. I don't know what it means to describe the mood of the city that people were looking for escapism in a nonpolitical parade. But, there it was. Next year it will be a few days before the midterm election and in 3 years a few days before the national election. Maybe then politics and political satire will reappear. We'll see. temp today 97.9

Journal of the Plague Years, Day 581. Yesterday I posted that nobody came to the parade dressed like Covid, but I was wrong. The FB page for Kostume Kult had two people with Covid costumes, scroll around and look for them. The costumes are kind of cute more than ominous so I'm not sure if these were in bad taste or demonstrated typical New York dark sarcastic humor. In any case, seeing these costumes from Kostume Kult colleagues (I camped with KK the last time at Burning Man) suggests maybe I was wrong and a Covid costume isn't that bad. Let other Facers reading this post give their opinions if they can find their way to Kostume Kults post and pictures. temp today 97.7

Journal of the Plague Year, Day 582. There wasn't a lot of new inside information I have that is better than the good news about new Covid treatments, but here is a revision of an old piece of good news. The residents at my ALF have been getting their booster shots this week and we have about 90% compliance. There also hasn't been a new case in months. The staff numbers are much less, but that's what happened when the vaccine originally came out. It took many months for the staff to come up to 90% and it might happen again. There also hasn't been a new covid case in the staff, as far as I know, so maybe they won't be reminded of the risk like they were last time. In any case, whether a big step for the residents or a small step for the staff, at least they were both in the right direction. temp today 98.3

Journal of the Plague Year, Day 585, Monday November 8. Let's start with some bad news and hope the week gets better. There has been a lot in the news about crime going up during covid, especially shootings and murders. This started in NYC before covid and accelerated during it. Now those crimes have leveled off or maybe gone down a little. What about little crimes? A little over a month ago one of the residents at my ALF was taking cash out of an ATM at a nearby super market and some guy came up and grabbed it out of her hand. He denied taking it to the store staff and the victim didn't want to go to the cops for fear of retribution. A few weeks ago another resident took money from an atm and it was pickpocketed out of her purse as she got on a bus. She is filling out a police report. The local bodega had it's glass door smashed and the cameras showed the person coming in and stealing two containers of detergent only. Three small crimes in a little over a month. I don't know if this is a trend or if it will continue, worsen, improve or what, but it's something to watch as covid improves. temp today 98.1

Journal of the Plague Year, Day 586. To stay on the dark side for another day, much of the violence and murder in the city recently has been blamed on people with mental illness. The theory is that covid related stress has made psychotic people more psychotic and tipped them into violence. At my facility I've posted that quarantine and covid related stress made many of our depressed patients and anxious patients even worse. But, we also have a few people with more problems like chronic schizophrenia and bi-polar disorder and stress hasn't made them more psychotic or violent. I think the message is that when supportive services are used, like at my place, mental illness can be relatively controlled even when stress for outside is increasing. Since the closing of large mental hospitals decades ago, community based treatments, especially residential facilities, have been inadequate. Those that operate do a reasonable job but their just aren't enough. I don't know how this is going to play out after covid, since there will still be an inadequate number of supportive housing facilities. But I hope some researcher can go back and study this problem before, during, and after covid so that when the next disaster occurs maybe we'll be ready for it. temp today 97.9

Journal of the Plague Year, Day 587. I think I previously posted that before covid vaccine was available, NPIs, Non-Pharmacological Interventions, were the only weapons we had. But not only did it help with covid, but ALL respiratory infections seemed to be drastically reduce. Flu went down 97%, instead of seeing 2-3 people a day with colds/coughs I saw virtually none the whole winter of 2020. I got no sinus infections (usually

2-3/winter), co-workers got no infections, my own doctor's patients got few infections, my pharmacy gave out almost no meds for respiratory infections. NPIs were very effective before the vaccine for all respiratory problems. Last week I saw two people on the same day that had coughs/respiratory infections. I'm worried about this. It's early in the winter and the peak of all these infections is only starting and all the NPIs from last year are not in place or strictly enforced. I hope we can keep some of the NPIs this winter, but they required discipline. I'm getting ready to continue with my mask everywhere for the next few months. Hope I can do it without weirding out my patients, friends, and family. temp today. 96.8

Journal of the Plague Year, Day 588. I recently poster about my patients getting their booster shots. I though it was 90% like the first two doses but I was told it was 75%. Like the post yesterday, I'm worried. I hope my patients and people in general don't get over confident. All of the non-vaccine precautions are slowly being decreased in high vaccine states, and being ignored or even banned in non-vaccine states. So far there is no new spike, but we still have about 1000 deaths a day, which means we'll be at about 800,000 by New Year's Day. I don't know what is happening with the staff, or younger people in general, but I wouldn't be surprised if those numbers are also less than the first two doses. Stay careful whenever possible. temp today 98.7

Journal of the Plague Year, Day 589. Does anything good come from epidemics? The Black Death may have finished off Feudalism and ushered in the Renaissance. This epidemic is raising workers salaries. Here's another little benefit. Because so many meetings are being held by Zoom instead of in person, we've gotten used to virtual presentations and virtual meetings. I applied to present a paper at a medical convention in March. It was rejected as a live presentation but accepted as a "On Demand" one. I'll have to put my presentation on slides and a video and that will be available on line. Most conventions have more requests to present than there is room for, but with videos like this many more people can present their work. This "hybrid" type meeting, some live some videos, has the potential for giving a lot of doctors, scientists, researchers, etc a chance to share their experience with others. I hope this continues and spreads to other organizations. I've got a lot of experience to share but not the time to write it up for medical journals. temp today 98.3

Journal of the Plague Years, Day 592, Monday November 15. While trying to monitor the city from the vantage point of riding under it in the subway, I've mentioned the emptiness of the Times Square subway station. A few weeks ago I thought it was picking up but I was probably wrong. In today's Daily News Harry Siegal described one of the weakest links in economic recovery. Office space. Before covid overall empty office space was about 10% but now it's 20% in Manhattan and 30% in midtown, including Times Square I think. Real estate value has dropped a lot with many more people working at home. The theaters are slowly opening, tourists are probably coming into the city a lot more, or will soon be coming in. But office workers not so much. This is very convenient for workers. Since bosses usually like to boss, having employees out of sight might not please them. But, that's what's happening, at least right now. There might be another aspect of remote working I hadn't thought of. Tune in tomorrow. temp today 98.0

Journal of the Plague Year, Day 593. What else might come out of remote working? The assisted living facility where I work was always 100% filled with a several month waiting list. The number of people dying or going to nursing homes was balanced by new people coming in. When covid hit and people didn't want to go to any facility, ALF or nursing home, we emptied out a little to now 85% occupancy. Again, discharges and admission have balanced out and we haven't gotten back up to full occupancy. People might still be afraid of institutions but our CEO had ad additional theory. Now that more people work at home they can care for a loved one and not have to use an ALF/nursing home to take care of them. Often families who were taking care of their oldest members couldn't do it because everyone had to go to work. Now that at least some people are home instead, they can take care of an elderly family member in a way that was impossible before. At least, that's a theory. If you read about this in the papers as a new trend, remember you heard it here first. temp today 98.1

Journal of the Plague Year, Day 594. Other posts on my main page today describe subway incidents of a guy masturbating and another eating his sweater, so this story will be relatively mild. Coming home today at 4, the train was packed and at the front of the car two large baby strollers among the standing crowd. But in the middle of the car was another stroller but with a dog in it. A cute white poodle, but still a dog in a stroller being pushed by a women whose mask was under her chin in a very crowded train. I know that police have their hands full watching for psychotics pushing people onto tracks and slashing people. I also know that my aunt, who took the subway every day from the Bronx down to the garment district to work, used to describe how flashers would cover themselves by holding a newspaper, looking around, and every once in a while lifting the paper to reveal their dicks. So, bizarre behavior isn't new. What I don't know is whether it's more frequent and more violent now that covid is stressing people, including psychotics. I hope someone does a study of this sometime soon so we can get a picture of how widespread covid damage is too all society and not just those who die from it. Tomorrow, more subway problems. temp today 98.3

Journal of the Plague Year, Day 595. When I take the subway in the morning, sometimes it's early about 8 and sometimes later at about 8:30. When I take it early I often see several people sleeping in the cars. Not sitting up, but lying down along the seats. I can't tell if these are psychotic homeless folks or just people who are homeless, but I have an idea. If they were just delusion mentally ill people you would see them all the time throughout the day since that type of behavior can strike at any time. But I don't think I've ever seen this behavior late in the day or at rush hour at 5, only very early in the morning. This makes me believe that these are simply people who are homeless, for whatever reason, and have been sleeping in the subways all night. I've read that 1-2,000 people fall into this category. I don't know if this is worse because of covid has pushed people into homelessness or less than before because covid relief has included an eviction moratorium. Maybe it just doesn't make a difference since homelessness has been bad in NYC for decades. When covid is over, or changed to just a routine annual winter plague like flu, we'll see if there is any difference. For now, I just observe and wonder. temp today 98.0

Journal of the Plague Year, Day 596. I recently had a covid related dream. Usually when I have a dream where I'm at work, it means it's time for a vacation. This dream was at work and I was sick and coughing. I remember holding up a bottle of cough syrup for myself, which I haven't actually done since the epidemic started, and getting ready to treat my cough. I've posted about how almost all winter coughs and colds disappeared when covid restrictions came in and I've posted about how relaxing these restrictions could bring them back, like the two patients who recently came to me with coughs. But this dream put me as one of the first people getting a new cold. I can, and have, written my own prescriptions for cold meds so maybe it's on my mind as I wait for it to hit me some time this winter. I hope it's just a dream and not a premonition. temp today 97.2

Journal of the Plague Years, Day 599, Monday November 22. There is some evidence in the mainstream press that there might be a little spike in covid occurring. At some point, I don't know when, covid might go from being a pandemic to endemic, from an unusual occurrence to something that is with us all the time, like the annual flu season. Other viruses like MERS and SARS came, spread, and then reduced to a low and maybe uncommon level. I hope covid does this, but if it doesn't it could change into a flu like season respiratory infection. The treatments will be the same with masks and isolation joining annual vaccines to keep the deaths to a relatively low level. This might take a few years to determine which path covid will take. I just hope the Tuesday Science Times has a better examination of this than the internet. temp today 97.6

Journal of the Plague Years, Day 600. In a few days I'll be going to a Thanksgiving dinner with some of my cousins. It's been a few years since I've had Thanksgiving dinner in person with family and this will be a nice getting back to normal moment. But, I'm still careful. I asked if everyone there will be vaccinated, and it looks like they all will be (lots of health care people and teachers all of whom are required to get vaccinated). Shopping for something to bring will be another return to normal with my usual places being boycotted (Rocco's on Bleeker street) or with lines that are already forming (Magnolia bakery). I'll get something somewhere, have a nice Zoom free get together, at least I hope it will be Zoom free, and eat and drink too much. But, carefully. There is another small spike in covid appearing and I don't want to go through this yet again. temp today 97.5

Journal of the Plague Years, Day 601. Yesterday I was a little worried about how my Thanksgiving get together would go, and how it would influence the future. Today I'm worried about how my patient's Thanksgiving will go. A while back residents of the facility had to show proof of a negative covid test when returning from a family visit. Before that there were virtually no family visits. Now all these restrictions are gone and people can visit freely. When a resident goes out with a family member there is a chance of person to person reinfection. But when they go out to dinner with an entire group of family members there might be a much higher chance. We can't track the status of every relative or the chances that they will infect our elderly frail residents. The positive side is that only about a half dozen residents are going to family for Thanksgiving, almost all the residents are vaccinated, and vaccinated patients who are re-infected with covid have a very small chance of a serious or deadly case. At least that's the way it has been up to now. We'll see if this Thanksgiving, and the upcoming holidays produce a worse outcome. We'll see by about February. temp today 98.1

Journal of the Plague Years, Day 606, Monday November 29. My snot is turning yellow. I know that I should have said "mucus" but it the midst of all this omicron news I had to do something to catch attention. I've posted about worrying that relaxing restrictions will make us vulnerable to the return of respiratory diseases, mild ones and deadly ones. Every years I got 2-4 sinus infections and colds except last year when there were none probably due to all the precautions we took. This mucus change is minor right now, maybe with a slight increase in clear runny noses and sneezes, but I don't know if this is a premonition of things to come in the next few months, or just a few bad days. (when I get omicron news that's not in the main media I'll let you know) temp today 97.9

Journal of the Plague Year, Day 607. While worrying about catching a bug yesterday, I thought about the Thanksgiving dinner I went to. About 15 people, including a half dozen kids. The adults were all vaccinated but I wasn't sure about the kids. They were all between 5 and 18 and so would qualify for vaccines by the new guidelines. They also all went to Catholic schools and had been required to wear masks. They were also all being required to get the shots but I'm not sure if they did yet. Catholic schools are strict and I don't think there have been any anti-mask or anti-v** protests at Catholic schools that I know of. Nuns are not know for their tolerance of non-compliance. In any case, no adults or kids were coughing or sneezing, so probably whatever this group was doing was probably working. But, I still get careful and obsessively observant when coughing, sneezing or blowing my nose. Let's see if I can make it through this winter without an infection. temp today 98.0

Journal of the Plague Year, Day 608. When this pandemic started the Department of Health (DOH) was very proactive. Every week they sent emails to me, as a physician, and several emails to the facility where I work. Information on the virus changed constantly and these emails changed guidelines constantly. But they can also be very, very slow. Hurricane Ida flooded the basement of our facility which produced extensive mold infestation. The mold was removed by ripping up the floor and walls of the basement offices. The mold is gone but so is the floor and some walls. Now we have to wait for DOH to give permission to replace the floors and walls. And we wait. And wait. It's frustrating to have needed work wait for a simple approval. This is why most assisted living facilities don't take Medicaid money because with Medicaid money comes Medicaid regulations and supervision. This isn't an anti-government rant since the benefit of Medicaid support is much better than the problems with it. But, I wish they would hurry just a little bit. temp today 97.3

Journal of the Plague Year, Day 609. After complaining about the DOH yesterday, I didn't want to give the impression that the rest of NY and US government weren't also screwing up at times. The basic rate for Medicaid and SSI pay to subsidize rents at our facility hasn't changed in many years. There have been individual grants and adjustments here and there but haven't been good enough to keep up with many increased costs over the years. What prevents this from becoming a typical right-wing "... see, government is the problem, not the solution..." or "...the government is all bad..." is the simple fact that without government subsidies, even poor ones, this program at our ALF would not even exist. This program, and one at The Village in the theater district (run by Village Care) are the only ones in Manhattan which accept Medicaid and without that help every assisted living facility in Manhattan that I know of would be cash only and very expensive. The city, state, and federal government make a lot of mistakes and sometimes can't deliver what's needed adequately, but without them many people, from the poorest to the richest, would be much much worse off. Government that governs least does not govern best. temp today 98.4

Journal of the Plague Year, Day 610. After a few days of ranting about government oversight of the facility I work in, what do we get for all of this? Before covid the main problems were keeping our residents healthy, alive, and out of the nursing home, which was often their biggest fear. Covid came in and it was bad at first. Two residents who had covid died in the hospital so we don't know if one of their previous conditions killed them, or covid did, or some combination. Other residents who got covid and died caught it in the hospital or rehab facility. Many residents and staff got covid and recovered without any obvious long term deficit. Our last known case of covid was in June. This can change at any time, but 6 months covid free, as far as we know, seems pretty good to us. So, whatever covid, omicron, or anything else does we'll be as ready as possible. I hope. temp today 97.9

Journal of the Plague Years, Day 613, Monday December 6 (a little late). Tonight I went to my first Christmas party of the year. Not a virtual party, a real in-person party. Fordham University had a party for some alumni who had donated over the years. It was at Cipriani's restaurant on 42nd street. It was fancy, but not black tie fancy. Good food, open bar (that's why this is a little late), and I saw a few friends but not too many. I graduated in 68 and most of my friends from Fordham are dead or scattered around the country. But, the party went well. Everyone was checked for vaccination cards and photo ID. Few attendees wore masks as we were constantly eating and drinking, but the staff was all masked and kept their mask on throughout the evening. The first part, but I hope not the last. Several more coming up soon. Let's hope the other parties are as compulsive about precautions so we don't have another covid spike as our New Year's gift. temp today 97.8

Journal of the Plague Years, Day 614. The NY Daily news letters to the editor column is entitled "Voice of the People" and it has a very wide range of letters from left and right political views, Yankees vs Mets fans, grass roots observations and complaints. There have been lots of letters about problems made worse by covid, like people sleeping in the subways, lack of mask enforcement, etc. Yesterday there was a regular article in The News about people sleeping in the subway. Those who have been following my posts know that many of these problems have been discussed here like subway mask enforcement and homelessness. I often end my posts with a prediction that what I write from an amateur grass roots posting level eventually ends up in the main stream media. The above issues are examples of this. There will be more. It takes time for info to get into the media, whether newspapers (for those who still read them) TV, internet, or whatever. There must be others posting about these issues but my internet search skills are poor. If you know of anyone else doing postings like mine, please let me know. It would be nice to have a whole accurate underground covid network that isn't filled with conspiracy theories, lies, and nonsense. temp today 97.2

Journal of the Plague Year, Day 615. In the mainstream media, medical journals, and internet we've been hearing about how un-vaccinated people can spread the disease, with illness and death a possible outcome. There's lower levels of discomfort. I just learned that the three or so residents who refused vaccines have prevented the facility from loosening up restrictions. Social distancing in the lobby and dining room must be maintained as long as anyone is un-vaccinated. The staff is now 100% vaccinated due to the state mandate, but residents can't be mandated to take the vaccine if they refuse. I'm not sure if this is explicit state regulations, facility policy, or some combination. There must be other places in the US where un-vaccinated people produce problems other than disease and death, like admissions to social gatherings or businesses. I just hope this Holiday season, when there will be tons of social gatherings, doesn't produce another peak in covid cases. temp today 97.1

Journal of the Plague Years, Day 616. I described one problem we were having at my ALF, today here's another. We are trying to get all staff and residents to weak masks in the facility when they are with anyone else.

Everybody complies most of the time except about 3-4 individuals. They all have some cognitive impairment and often get upset when reminded about the mask. Since everyone else is masked and almost everyone in the building is vaccinated, a few people without masks won't make a major difference. The problem is that this situation as minor as it is, is persistent. Having a small number of maskless people and a small number of unvaccinated people presents a low level of risk. But, we don't know what's coming. Will there be another spike soon, since some numbers in NYC are turning bad? Will omicron be bad or will the next one after omicron be bad? As trivial as these problems appear, we'll only be safe when everything is as close to zero as we can get. temp today 98.3

Journal of the Plague Years, Day 617. Here is another post on the partial reopening of NYC. About two weeks ago on a Saturday night I went to Cafe Katja on Orchard for dinner and they were closed for a private event. This week on both Tuesday and Thursday night there were private events at Piccolo Angolo on Hudson. These are the first large scale private parties I'm aware of so I'm taking it as a good sign. I don't mind being locked out of my favorite restaurants if it's in the name of increasing their business and, presumably, their survival. It also indicates we might be getting safer in crowds of moderate size. On the other had, Mt Sinai Geriatrics department and Vista on 5th assisted living are both having Christmas parties remotely, no person to person contact. Well, you win some and you lose some. Time might make this better, omicron might make this worse. We'll see. temp today 97.0

Journal of the Plague Years, Day 620, Monday December 13. On Saturday night I got together with friends from graduate school at Lehman college in The Bronx. It's a get together we have a few times a year at various restaurants around NYC, and this time it was in Bronxville in Westchester at Bistro 143. The dinner and drinks were good and it was good to see my friends again. But, when I went in and reached for my vaccine card the manager said not to. No need for ID in Westchester. I forget if we were required to wear masks before seating. Most of the staff did but I'm not sure if they all did. Variations like this, from town to town makes me nervous. Lots of people commute from Westchester into NYC every day. I'm not sure if the spike in covid that appears to be happening is because of this variation in rules, the remaining anti-v******, omicron, or whatever. I hope some day some epidemiologist will tease out these different factors and tell us what's the most important. This might help us when the next epidemic comes, and there will be more epidemics in the future. temp today 97.7

Journal of the Plague Years, Day 621. With a new spike in covid just starting, the state is requiring masks for all indoor activities that don't require vaccine ID cards. Many of the small places I've gone to, like take out stores, already have signs requesting masks. But, I'm not sure which new places will comply. I've already heard of a few places in the suburbs not complying, but it's still only two days of this new rule. It might take me time to collect anecdotal evidence myself, so I'll ask any of the Facers reading my post to chime in as they hear of places complying or not complying. Let's see how this new rule is going. Remember, a new spike is starting, so this isn't just an academic exercise, unfortunately. temp today 97.6

Journal of the Plague Years, Day 622. Let's switch to more positive items. Last weekend Santacon returned to NYC. An in person bar crawl involving thousands of people dressed in various Santa Claus costumes. In previous years it had gotten pretty drunken and raucous to the point where some bars wouldn't let them in. This year, so far, no reports of really bad behavior. Maybe because people weren't up to acting like jerks, maybe because every bar and restaurant was being more careful about ID given covid precautions, maybe something else. Send in you suggestions. In any case, a tradition has returned and NYC is one step closer to normal, or at least to "normal" for NYC. temp today 98.0

Journal of the Plague Years, Day 623. One way NYC is coming back is the reopening of old businesses. But there's also the appearance of new businesses. Last Saturday the weather was great and Bleecker street was packed with people window shopping and really shopping. Many new stores whose brands I never heard of have opened there this year. There was one place call Ring Concierge with lots of jewelry and a line of about a dozen people in front. I don't know if it was a sale, a new hot brand, or what but they had a line when Magnolia bakery across the street didn't. I wish these new stores well even though I'll never shop in any of them. More NYC resiliency. Also, the day after an internet search for Ring Concierge its ads started showing up on this FB page. I recently searched Magnolia bakery and the next day its ads started popping up. With all this internet exposure I'm not sure why people have to line up in front of an actual store, but I guess anything to produce a buzz is worth it. temp today 98.4

Journal of the Plague Years, Day 624. I've posted about NYC resiliency for the city, city businesses and new start up businesses. What about the people of NYC and their response. The media has a lot of articles about people coming into the city, whether returning ex-patriots or newbies and the hot apartment rental market. Here is something a lot smaller. When coming back from dinner Saturday night I passed through the Times Square subway station about 10 PM and in the area where musicians play there was a small band playing rock music. They were playing "I'm a Believer". In the 60s (yes, that far back), a band called the Monkees was popular, although not with me. But, it was well known, had a run of popularity and is a cultural reference for boomers of my generation. Last week Mike Nesmith one of the band members, died. There were brief obituaries and some of us remembered him. I thought this tribute, in a subway station on a Saturday night was a melancholy comment of how life goes on. Even in the middle of a pandemic, which isn't over yet, there is still a moment here or there for a joyful reminder of things we have had, and enjoyed, over the years. I dropped a buck in their collection box, as I often do, and walked by, but for some reason this simple tune from a long gone group just cheered me up as I returned to the real world. temp today 98.7

Journal of the Plague Years, Day 627, Monday December 20. There has been a lot of mainstream media attention to people getting covid testing. Last week I saw the same thing but didn't post it so I could do an uplifting piece on Friday. But, this is what I saw. Coming across 23rd street after going to my bank I saw a line of about a dozen people outside a City MD storefront. This wasn't surprising since I saw the same at the start of the plague. What was new was that some of the little sidewalk tents that do testing also had lines in front, at a few locations on Sixth avenue. I don't know if it's just fear of omicron, or to be safe for family holiday get togethers, or to be safe to travel. But the mainstream media wasn't just hyping the situation, it actually is happening on the street. For how long? Who knows? temp today 98.4

Journal of the Plague Years. At the 110th street Central Park North subway station I was amazed this morning. There were 5 cops, all wearing masks. One of them appeared to have written a ticket to a guy who wasn't wearing a mask. I didn't get too close but the guy was holding a paper the size of a summons and the cop was closing his summons book. I've posted about the lack of enforcement of mask mandates but this was the first clear evidence that an enforcement does sometimes take place. I was surprised and also pleased that this current omicron panic is maybe producing some practical effect. Maybe it was just a one day happening, but now I'll be looking more carefully. We really don't need a fifth wave of covid deaths. temp today 97.5

Journal of the Plague Years, Day 629 (yesterday was 628 but I forgot to label it). An internet web site said that my zip code 10014 had the highest covid positive rate in NYC, 16.4%. Not trusting the internet I went to nyc.gov website and looked up a Covid map which confirmed this. 10014 last week had about 16.4% people tested positive. Why my neighborhood? Well, I've posted a lot about the crowds of people in restaurants and bars all over my area. Many were wearing masks but when crowds are very big it might not be enough. Who knows how many places were bending the rules, such as Rocco's pastry shop on Bleecker. Now we will have to see if death rates a few weeks from now follow this pattern. Breaking the rules kills people, and it might kill people again. Sad. temp today 98,6

Journal of the Plague Year, Day 629 Addendum. One of the talking heads on MSNBC reminded me of another explanation of the high covid count in 10014. This is a very wealthy area where people can afford to wait on line for a few minutes or hours to get a test. People in poorer areas, which is virtually the whole city, have less flexibility. Whether or not this matters and whether or not the rest of the city will catch up to us, only time will tell.

Journal of the Plague Years, Day 630. With the spike in omicron/covid people are worried that a new shut down might be ordered. But some damage might be already happening. Last week I went to one of my favorite restaurants and was told that almost 70 out of 70 reservations for a Saturday night got cancelled. Another favorite said that reservations weren't being made in the first place. Another restaurant said business was down but not a disaster yet, and a pastry shop had slightly less walk in customers. I don't know if these few cases indicate a trend, but there is a chance that people will stay away from night life like this for a while. On the other hand, all these places were still being careful about vaccine cards and ID. We'll see how this plays out in the next few weeks to months. temp today 99.7

Journal of the Plague Years, Day 631. Last week on both the Rachel Maddow show and in a letter from the NY DOH there was a graph showing new covid cases in nursing homes. Unvaccinated patients had a big increase in case, double vaccinations had a moderate increase, and vaccinations plus boosters had no increase. I haven't been able to find the graph to show, because it is a very stark reminder that sometimes these interventions work, and work very well, even among the sickest and most debilitated populations. That's about the best news we have right now. Better news would be when the rest of the country realizes this and everyone gets the vaccines and boosters before the present omicron/covid spike gets much worse. temp today 99.1

Journal of the Plague Years, Day 634, Monday December 27th. You may have noticed on last weeks posts that I had temperatures of 99.7 and 99.1. Normally these low temps would mean nothing but with the worry about covid I felt it would be negligent not to be a little more compulsive than normal. I found a local testing place, ZoomCare365 on Carmine street. It looked like a pop-up storefront with curtains instead of rooms but I got the test. They didn't call or email me with the results, which was annoying, so I walked by down there on Christmas morning and they printed out my negative result. I went and had a Christmas meal with my cousins with one less worry. Hypervigilance like this might be with us for a while. temp today 98.8

Journal of the Plague Years, Day 635. Guidelines or mandates for vaccines and quarantine are getting more complicated. Let's take vaccines first. It's becoming clearer that getting the third shot, the booster, increases immunity a lot. Details vary from study to study but "a lot" covers them all. In my ALF facility 85% of residents and 30% of staff have gotten the booster. Both these numbers are better than the national average for long term care facilities, including I believe, nursing homes where they really need higher numbers. It would really help if both these numbers were closer to 100% but it will take time to do that, just like it took time to get the two shot vaccination rates up. It might even take a few people getting sick before the rest are frightened into getting the boost. I'll try to get quarantine guidelines figured out, but that seems a little more complicated as we'll see tomorrow. temp today 98.7

Journal of the Plague Years, Day 636. One area of confusion about covid is the question of quarantines. The CDC recently shortened the quarantine period from 10 to 5 days for healthcare workers and some others. There are lots of details and exclusions. The facility where I work still requires 14 days of quarantine for anyone exposed to covid. The difference is because of different needs, goals, and environments. CDC had to at least consider the need to get people back to work, and after 5 days an active case of covid is much less infectious. Other people are much less likely to get it. Healthcare workers contact lots of sick people every day and to be much more cautious with them is understandable. After the catastrophe in nursing homes, the DOH is also much more cautious, going beyond what the science proves or what the economy needs. Patients in nursing homes, hospitals, and ALFs are monitored more closely than the general public but a virtually a captive audience when it comes to testing and treatment. People in the general population when faced with 14 days isolation, or even 10 days, may simply avoid getting tested and remain hidden. For all diseases, people who might be sick avoid going to a doctor or ER if the consequences are too severe. That's one of the reasons why paid sick days are so important, so that sick people don't bring their illness into work with them rather than lose pay. That's just the way it is. If the CDC guidelines were too harsh and people didn't get tested the true level of covid infections and deaths might remain hidden. So, we'll see how this works out. It's not so confusing once you know the details, but there are a lot of details and people often want simple one size fits all explanations. I wish medicine, and life in general, was that simple. temp today 97.8

Journal of the Plague Year, Day 637. Tomorrow I'll be eating and drinking, so no posting. But, I'll try and have my good news post today. When riding on the subway this morning there was a big guy standing next to me in front of the door to get off at the next stop. He was a few inches taller than me, in his 30s, with gym shorts of some type and I think a gym bag. A real healthy looking shtarker. Then my allergies, which I've had every winter since moving back from California 30 years ago, kicked in and I took out my handkerchief and blew my nose. Slowly the guy moved down the car to the next door to get out that way, which was a longer walk for him to the station exit. Just from blowing my nose! Next time I'm going to try a fake sneeze or cough and see if I can get him running. To think it is so easy to protect yourself on the subway just with a few sniffles. I wonder if I can use it to get a seat? temp today 96.9

Journal of the Plague Years, Day 641, Monday Jan 3 2022. Recently, the city started requiring all small businesses to get vaccinations for full time and part time employees. I didn't realize how far reaching this was until I got a notice from the company that manages my co-op. All full time employees covers the doormen, super, and janitor but part-time covers people coming in to provide services like home health aides, housekeepers, tutors, repair people, etc. For all of them, they have to have proof of vaccination and the individual co-op owner has to make a copy and keep it. I don't know how this is going to be enforced for every apartment house in NYC or what the penalties will be, but it seems to cover a lot of people. So if you worry about small businesses being effected, it will also include of lot of individuals and their helpers. I hope this helps a little. Temp today 98.9

Journal of the Plague Years, Day 642. Speaking of small businesses, last Thursday, New Years Eve eve, I was walking back home and arrived at Hudson Street for dinner. My favorite place was completely closed, which was pretty strange since it's never closed on Thursdays. As I walked down Hudson I saw many restaurants/bars almost completely empty or closed. Usually packed places like the White Horse and Dante's were half filled. Why? First I thought that too many customers cancelled reservations due to omicron/covid fear and some closed for that reason. A few weeks ago I posted about the cancellation epidemic.

Then I thought maybe some had staff members who tested positive or were sick and they didn't have the people to open. In either case, it was bleak on a normally business night. If I figure it out I'll let you know. What about New Years Eve? Tomorrow for that news. temp today 96.9

Journal of the Plague Years, Day 643. My plans for New Years Eve was to go to the National Arts Club with some friends, who are members there for dinner and then to the Lower East Side for Midnight. The NAC is an upscale place, traditional, on Gramercy Park. But when most of their reservations were cancelled, presumably due to covid/omicron fear, the dinner was cancelled. The Lower East Side was more determined. Lamia's Fish Market on Avenue B, whose owners I know, persisted. A few of us went down there, showed our vaccination cards and hung out until the ball dropped at midnight. The crowd was younger, noisier, sexier clothing and with a more downtown/LES vibe. It was fun. But I couldn't help but notice they did have some empty tables in some of their smaller rooms. The four of us had a room for twelve to ourselves. On a normal Friday night I'm pretty sure this place would be packed. So, covid didn't shut them, but it probably hurt them. When I asked Lamia how they were doing, she said "we're trying to survive". I hope they, and all the empty places on Hudson, do survive. temp today 98.9

Journal of the Plague Years, Day 644. I spoke to one of the owners of a restaurant that was closed last week when I walked down half empty Hudson street. Several members of the staff had gone to a family get together but later found out that the other family members were not vaccinated and that covid/omicron had swept through the family. The restaurant people did the only ethical thing and all got tested for covid, all were negative, and the restaurant reopened. Omicron is different than Delta. Delta moves slowly. Several branches of my family have been hit with Omicron and in the course of a week more than half the family was infected. If just one person with Omicron comes into a family gathering the entire family can be infected amazingly fast. This is especially true if the first person is asymptomatic. In my family, so far, no deaths, but others haven't been that lucky. Get vaccinated, wear masks, do everything you can do to not be that infectious first case (and I don't mean colloidal silver, ivermectin, or chloroquine). If your infection kills a loved one, it will haunt you for the rest of your life with survivors guilt. As a geriatrician I've had patients deeply remorseful about things they did decades ago. It shouldn't be this hard to help people avoid a deadly disease. temp today 99.3

Journal of the Plague Years, Day 645. On previous posts, I've bragged about how precautions for covid helped eliminate other respiratory diseases. For all of 2020 and almost all of 2021 I saw almost no respiratory diseases in my practice, and my own primary care doctor and local pharmacy confirmed this. Around the end of November 2021 this stopped. I started to see a few pneumonias, bronchitis attacks, coughs, colds, sore throats, etc. Yesterday, my turn came. I got up with a few coughs and a little phlegm, which normally means nothing. By the time I was in work I had a runny nose, more coughing more phlegm but no temp. I saw the patients I had to see and left early before I got worse. All last night coughing, congested, temp of 100.2 this morning, when I stayed home instead of going to my practice. I don't know if I caught it at the big New Years Eve party, the subways, work, or whatever, but I clearly have the same cold that I've been getting for the last 30 years when I moved back to NYC from LA. We've been slowly relaxing a lot of the precautions for covid and it was only a matter of time before every other respiratory bug took notice. So, cough syrup, lozenges,, chicken soup, etc until this passes. Antibiotics if it really gets bad. But there is good news, for "Good News" Friday. I tested negative for covid by the pcr test a few days ago. That really would have been a problem. temp today 100.1

Journal of the Plague Years, Day 648, Monday January 10. I'm still trying to investigate what's happening with respiratory diseases of all types right now. I was at one of my dentists office today and he said he saw no increase in colds/coughs, but an increase in people cancelling appointments because of covid contacts or possible cases. My pharmacist has noticed that all the cough syrups have sold out and the suppliers and manufacturers have new supplies on back orders that are lasting until February or even March. Whether there is a shortage in the supply chain or whether there is increased demand scooping up supplies as they come in isn't clear. The worry isn't just about covid. From the first outbreak in 2020 there has been a worry that if covid and seasonal diseases (flu, pneumonia, colds, etc) both peak at the same time the medical system will be super stressed and deaths will increase. The last two years seasonal diseases decreased as I've reported. This year might not follow the pattern. The regular diseases and covid, even a possibly milder omicron, might both peak at the same time. There's no telling how bad or how routine those peaks will be, and we won't know for another month or two. temp today 97.5

Journal of the Plague Years, Day 649. Some time at the start of the plague, the NY DOH offered tests for covid to ALFs like mine. About a hundred people signed up, a mix of residents and staff, and every one was negative. Last week the DOH made the same offer and about 100 people got the test. Ten were positive, 6 residents and 4 staff. Most were asymptomatic, although a few might be mildly ill. None went to the hospital so far. This is the difference between the original alpha strain, the delta strain, and the omicron. It travels fast and can often spread quickly before the first case, or even a random test, indicates its presence. Our facility is now on lockdown with everyone quarantined in their rooms, all meals and meds delivered, no group activities, more PPE for staff, etc. Individual trips outside the building or individual family member visits are still allowed, but discouraged whenever possible. We are trying to figure how aggressively to treat the mildly ill patients (to the ER or not?). This coming Friday the DOH is back again for another round of testing. This disease is changing from month to month, but it's not letting up. temp today 97.6

Journal of the Plague Years, Day 650. I mentioned yesterday that 6 residents and 4 staff were positive for covid, out of a total of about 100 tested. It was too long a post to go into significance, but here it is. The race we now have is between more covid deaths because omicron is spreading rapidly vs less death because omicron might be less deadly. But there are reports from all over the world on both sides of the argument. It hasn't sorted out yet with enough data. But that hasn't stopped people from speculating and it hasn't stopped critics from saying that scientists don't know what they are saying. That's an excuse for doing nothing. The data we do have still shows that getting vaccinated and boosted dramatically decreases the death rate from covid. We can criticize every variation from every study, but it doesn't change what should be done. Get the vaccines and boosts now, before it's made mandatory (like, I think some businesses in France) and there's a rush. temp today 98.3

Journal of the Plague Years, Day 651. Yesterday I suggested that everyone get the third shot booster before it becomes mandatory. Today I got an email from Mt. Sinai, where I am a voluntary attending faculty member. It was warning its workers to prepare for a mandatory booster requirement from the state. The data is slowly becoming strong enough to show the value of a booster and so the state is on the verge of a requirement. This is inconvenient for a lot of people and will piss off a lot of anti-v****** and vaccine skeptics. Too bad. We have to be determined to do everything we can to make us all safer while the Supreme Court seems to be doing every thing it can to make us less safe. Sad. 98.2

Journal of the Plague Years, Day 652. To keep Friday on a good news track, I'm trying to find some grass roots report I can give.

Well, with 10 recent positive covid tests at my ALF and another few for our hospital patients, none have died. I hesitate to brag about this since it could change in a day, but let's take it while we can. Also, some NYC date shows that covid cases and deaths here in the city have started to go down. With so many other cases statewide and national this gets lost in the larger bad news. Maybe in a few weeks the national numbers will start to go down like NYC's, assuming NYC numbers are real and not a blip in the curve. Sorry, that's the best I can do today. Maybe next week will be better. temp today 97.8

Journal of the Plague Years, Day 656, Tuesday January 18th. My cousin Bonnie Fogler died last week. If you can get to her posts on FB or read her book "The Other Side of Healing" you can see what type of person she was. Her posts were always positive and uplifting, and her book told how strong family support and spirituality helped her through medical problems in the past. But that wasn't enough this time, and after a hospitalization, in which she fought as best she could, she passed last week. Because of the various quarantines in NY and New Jersey, we hadn't seen each other in person in a few years, although we spoke on the phone and through FB. I'll miss her. temp today 97.9

Journal of the Plague Years, Day 657. After my sad post from yesterday I tried looking for something more positive, and decided to settle for something that's at least not very negative. Last week my ALF did covid testing again and 7 residents and one staff member out of about 125 tests was positive. The week before it was 10 out of 100 (6 residents and 4 staff). So in about 2-3 weeks 13 residents out of a patient population of about 110 came back positive. There are probably others that are covid positive but refused testing. How is this a positive finding? None of the residents or staff were very sick, none went to the hospital for covid related illness (although some did for other reasons), and nobody died. The omicron strain moves very fast, more than the original alpha strain or delta. But on a national and local level it doesn't appear as lethal, especially for those who have been vaccinated or boosted, as many of the staff and residents at my place have been. That's not the best news, which would be no positive tests, but it's relatively good. Tomorrow we test again, so eventually we'll see if this has maxed out, still expanding, or what. temp today 97.6

Journal of the Plague Years, Day 658. You can see from my posts about covid tests at my ALF, covid can spread really fast. Last Thursday I was reminded how easy it is to make a mistake and spread it. I had a reunion with several people who used to work at the ALF who I hadn't seen in a few years. I got a lift up to the Bronx (the driver is in this FB group, so take a bow if you want) and after a frustrating hour in traffic we got up to Arthur Avenue and Emilia's restaurant. I was really happy to see my friends. It wasn't until the middle of the dinner that I realized that we hadn't been vaccine carded when we went in. Maybe the host who was a regular there told them we were all ok. Maybe because it was The Bronx (to paraphrase the movie Chinatown, "Forget it Jake, it's the Bronx). Maybe this was a place that just didn't card people. If I realized this when I entered, I probably would have gone in any way rather than miss this occasion but I would have been nervous, at least until the first glass or two of wine. Of the 7 of us, 4 were retired and probably vaccinated, me and one other are in health care and definitely vaccinated, and one was a college professor and probably vaccinated. I'm not sure about the restaurant staff. That was last Thursday. I haven't heard of any of us getting sick, and I had another covid test today at work. We probably all were lucky but it's so easy to make a mistake. temp today 98.2

Journal of the Plague Years, Day 659. A few weeks ago a wave of 10 new covid cases occurred in my ALF (where I work, not where I live) and we went into complete shut down. No group activities, everyone stayed in their rooms while food and meds were brought to them. This is how we controlled the alpha strain at the start of this plague. The ALF administrators looked at our policies and new guidelines from the CDC and NY DOH and now we have a more open policy. Individuals who test positive have to be on this type of isolation, but everyone negative doesn't. Un-infected residents can now go up to the beautiful dining room for meals, patients can congregate in the activity room and lobby, and come to the Wellness Center for their meds. Quarantine makes people depressed, anxious, weak, severely isolated and just plain miserable. I hope this more open policy can last. We did a bunch of testing yesterday and the results will be back in a few days. I expect a few more residents and staff will be positive and almost all will not be very sick. I hope this open policy, instead of 2020's complete quarantine can be maintained. Surviving covid is important but having some quality of life while you do it is also important. temp today 98.4

Journal of the Plague Years, Day 662, Monday January 24. In times of stress, people sometimes resort to comfort food. What about comfort music? Last night I was having dinner at Cafe Katja on Orchard street. They usually have a very eclectic selection of music playing as background, but last night they had oldies. First, "Fortunate Son" by Creedance Clearwater Revival (1969) a song linked to the Viet Nam war so closely that it was satirized on The Family Guy. The "Rudi" by the Specials (79) and several others I forgot. When I went over to Cafe Palermo on Orchard street I was treated to Fats Domino, Everly Brothers, Buddy Holly, and Little Anthony and the Imperials. The exact songs don't matter. You get the picture. I felt nostalgic and very much at ease. Comfort music. By the time I got to The Left Bank on Perry street, they were playing modern music that I didn't recognize or particularly care about. Times of stress, like epidemics, bring out a yearning for simpler foods, simpler music and simpler times. I wonder if future generations will look back at 2022 the same nostalgic way. 97.7

Journal of the Plague Years, Day 663. I've posted about observations in the subway to reflect what's going on above ground. Now I'll address what's going on below ground. On each of the last four days I've seen cops in the subways. Twice on 14th street and twice at 119th street. They weren't giving out tickets for no masks, they were standing and watching people. They were also all wearing masks, a new development. This might be good in that it shows the city is ramping up protection from violence in the subways. It might also be bad since it shows the protecting is needed on an increasing basis. It might take a few month to see if there actually is a change in subway crime, especially violence or psychotic behavior. Meanwhile, some city council members like Erik Bottcher, my councilperson, are trying to expand mental health services so that this problem can be addressed by increased caring and not just increased cops. We'll see which approach is working, but meanwhile we are trying them both. temp today 98.5

Journal of the Plague Year, Day 664. How slow can you go? A few weeks ago we had 10 positive covid tests. The next week we had 7. Last week we had three, although only 90 people were tested. This is slowly decreasing, but very slowly. The good news is that there have been no hospitalizations or deaths, but that is probably because almost everyone is vaccinated and most are booster. Nationally, deaths are over 2000 a day because so many people are unvaccinated. Not only is this death rate terrible, and preventable, but it enables the virus to continue floating around in the population for longer and longer periods. We are not stuck with this virus just because it is so resilient, but also because we are so inconsistent. I just hope we somehow break out of this pattern before the next mutation comes along. A mutant that spreads as fast as omicron but is as deadly as alpha or delta would set us back 2 years and could kill hundreds of thousands more. temp today 98.1

Journal of the Plague Years, Day 665. Since these cases of covid/omicron seem to be lasting for ever, has there been any progress in the last two years? At my facility, in the start of the pandemic we had about 15 cases out of 227 residents and staff. Recently, we've had about 20 cases out of about 215 residents and staff. It looks like things are worse. But just because something is happening more frequently, doesn't mean it's worse. Of the original 15 cases about a dozen went to the hospital or rehab and came back to us, but two died. Of the 20 recent cases none went to the hospital and none died. A more frequent mild disease is not worse than a less frequent deadly disease. During an average winter there are even a larger number of colds/coughs that don't require hospitalization. Maybe some day covid will be as harmless as typical colds or even flu cases, but not yet. temp today 97.4

Journal of the Plague Year, Day 666. No clear good news on this ominously numbered date, but maybe some theoretically good news. When William Jenner and many others noticed that cowpox protected milkmaids from smallpox, it's use for vaccines took off. Anti-****** now think that a natural immunity like that one will protect them and they don't need no stinkin' vaccines. Natural immunity from a mild case of omicron covid, as described in some of my posts and the main stream media, helps a little. But natural immunity, vaccinations, and boosters (and whatever comes next) will help a lot more. Why have one protection against a deadly disease when you can have many. We don't tell our patients that if they exercise they will decrease the chances of a heart attack, we tell them to exercise, and maintain normal weight, and maintain normal cholesterol, and maintain normal blood pressure. For some diseases, like measles, a single infection can give long term complete immunity, but not covid. I don't know what else to say to save the lives of people taken in by anti-v***** propaganda. Well, maybe "Good Luck" would be appropriate. temp today 98.0

Journal of the Plague Years, Day 669, Monday January 31. A while back I posted about going to dinner in the Bronx on Arthur Avenue, where I grew up, but not noticing that the restaurant didn't ask for vaccine cards. Maybe the host vouched for us and they thought it wasn't needed, but who knows? A friend just told me that he went for dinner on City Island and again they didn't ask for vaccination cards. I knew Staten Island is being thick headed and reckless about covid, but I didn't know it had spread to The Bronx. Maybe it's just any borough outside of Manhattan figures the city isn't paying attention to them and so they can do what they want. Maybe the health inspectors haven't gotten to them yet, but soon will. In any case, people are still being careless. How many have to get sick and die before we stop being careless? temp today 98.1

Journal of the Plague Years, Day 670. If the city is having a hard time enforcing vaccine ID mandates in the city's restaurants and bars, I have a suggestion. Fining them isn't enough even when you do inspect them and catch them breaking the rules. Some of the Village restaurants are paying rents in the tens of thousands every month so a fine of one thousand or even five thousand can just be added to the overheard. There's one thing that can't be shrugged off so easily. Dock their letter grade. Restaurants are very proud and loud whenever they get an A rating. If that rating goes down to B in a neighborhood with many A places it could do real long term damage to a place. And if the grade went to a C that could make the difference between surviving and not. I usually take the side of small businesses, and this punishment might seem harsh, but so is covid, and death. temp today 98.0

Journal of the Plague Years, Day 671. More on covid enforcement. About 4,000 NYC employees will soon be fired if they don't vaccinate. The a little over 1% of the total NYC employees. In other words, almost 99% of NYC employees are willing to get vaccinated. Mandates by their employer, NYC, might annoy them or really infuriate them, but they are complying. I normally take the side of employees vs bosses but not this time. Again, and how many times need we say this, mandating vaccinations are aimed at protecting us from a deadly disease. It doesn't matter that it's going down right at this minute since it can bounce back at any time, as it has done FOUR times. Every precaution, masks, distancing, isolation, vaccines, boosters, or whatever comes next, should be used to fight this. We're approaching 900,000 dead. I don't know where the 4,000 will go, but good luck to them. temp today 97.7

Journal of the Plague Years, Day 672. After posting about city workers losing their jobs for anti-v** behavior, here's some comparison with the health care field. All health care workers in NY State must get vaccinated and boosted or lose their jobs. Very simple. Before covid, everyone got flu shots or wore a mask if there was a medical reason they couldn't take it. The comparison between city vs health workers seems lopsided since health workers see a lot of sick people and cops/firemen etc only see a few (along with seeing each other). But what makes the two groups comparable is that they are being asked to do something that is very simple. Vaccines are very effective and have side effects that are less common than side effects of virtually any medication there is, including aspirin. Vaccines are easy. Mandates occur in virtually every job at some time or another. Why this mandate is unacceptable makes no sense. temp today 98.1

Journal of the Plague Years, Day 673. For about the last month I've been posting about testing being done at the assisted living where I work. At first, there were 10 positives, then about 7, then 3. This week about 95 were tested and zero were positive. Finally, a little good news. Of course we know that good news sometimes doesn't last long. Just one infected person can spread covid through out the ALF. Just one neighborhood of anti-v****** can spread it through a city or state. And just one more new variant or mutant can spread it through the country or world. But, let's take what we can get while we can get it. Zero positives! Good news. temp today 98.2

Journal of the Plague Years, Day 676, Monday Feb 7th. I usually don't just post on something retorted someplace else, but today's an exception to that rule. In the New England Journal of Medicine issue of January 27 there was a report of covid vaccination rates in nursing homes. They looked at nursing homes in areas with high numbers of covid cases. Those homes with staffs that had a low level of vaccinations, there were more cases of covid among staff and residents and more deaths among residents.

Lack of vaccinated staff killed the residents they were caring for and made everyone sicker. This isn't a surprise since similar data was found for flu vaccine results in nursing homes. Staff who don't get vaccinated are infectious and can kill people. How does this effect my ALF? Tune in tomorrow. temp today 98.7

Journal of the Plague Years, Day 677. So, how do you get something out of a medical journal, posted yesterday, down into the trenches where we are. At my ALF it is simple. All staff are vaccinated and boosted by the end of this week. A handful of residents with severe immune deficiencies are getting their FOURTH vaccination this week. And of the 104 residents of the facility 84 have gotten a booster on top of their two vaccinations. We are still working on the other 20 residents to see if we can convince more of them to take the booster. Because covid numbers have been going down recently, some people think this is the time to lay back and take it easy. I think these numbers give us a breather that we can use to double down on everything possible, especially vaccines. We don't know how low covid numbers will go, or if they might rebound if they find a reservoir among the unvaccinated, or even a reservoir among deer and other wildlife (according to the NY Times Science section today). Don't let up, at least not right now. temp today 98.7

Journal of the Plague Years, Day 678. Today my ALF admitted its first new admission in many months. One new admission does not constitute a trend, but months without an admission does constitute a trend, and a very bad one. so, what does this mean? You want to see small businesses surviving, but why an ALF? There is a shortage of housing for low income elderly and so any ALF stays open can help with this problem. Most people, including myself, think that keeping a person in their own homes is best, but sometimes this just isn't possible. ALFs of all types can provide services that often families cannot provide. Also, families are now able to re-enter the work force and not spend extended periods of time caring for their loved ones who have problems that are beyond their abilities. ALF transfer is voluntary, but when you need one, you really need one. This one admission, if we're lucky, might be the first step in making this service increasingly available to elderly and their families who need it. temp today 98.0

Journal of the Plague Years, Day 679. At the start of the plague, one of the ways I kept track of its effect on the city was to count taxis and compare the empty ones to occupied ones. If I remember correctly (and I'm not going back through 600 posts to find out) the empty to fill ratio was about two or three to one. So many empty taxis. Last night while having dinner in a Hudson Street restaurant, I did some more counting. There were 47 occupied taxis and 22 empty ones. The ratio had flipped. Since NYC resilience is a recurring theme of these posts, it made me happy to see this, since the opposite numbers would have gotten me depressed. Take good news where you can get it, even on Hudson street. temp today 97.7

Journal of the Plague Year, Day 680. The vaccinations continue. Ten more residents boosted bringing us up to about 94 out of 104. there are a few that will always refuse, but we're getting pretty close to 100%. This is about the most we can do without a total lockdown, which is out of the question right now. I'll make this short tonight because there's not much better news I can post other than more people getting safe. temp today 98.1

Journal of the Plague Years, Day 683, Monday Feb 14th. Yesterday, as I was walking over to Orchard street for dinner I passed a young guy in the street talking on his phone. I am so used to wearing a face mask I even do it on the street when I don't have to. I swear I heard him say into his phone "we should shame these people who keep wearing masks" or something like that. Well, pardon me for not taking advice from a brain dead Millennial but when I have to decide between being extra cautious, especially when walking through streets packed with maskless folks eating, drinking and talking loudly, or playing around with a disease that's killed almost 900,000 of us, I opt for caution. If I heard him right, and I really hope I didn't, I couldn't help to wonder what would make somebody think this. Are masks just "uncool" and so 2021? Is it because talking heads on you know what network undermine masks, vaccines or anything else that helps? If some kid walking along the street were and isolated case, I could laugh this off, but it's stuff like this is keeping this epidemic going and going. temp today 98.3

Journal of the Plague Years, Day 684. A follow up to previous posts. After much controversy NYC finally let go about 1400 employees (less than 0.5% of its workforce) who refused to get vaccinated. As much as I hate to see workers get fired, I also don't like to see workers spread deadly and preventable diseases. The city won't suffer from a loss of 1400. Maybe some will change their minds in their next jobs, though I doubt it. By the way, those who refused were not classified as "fired" but as "quit". I don't know all the details of labor law, but if your job description changes (with the approval of the union that holds your contract) and you refuse, can this be considered a voluntary quitting? I guess so unless these guys sue and get a friendly judge. Some red states are giving unemployment benefits to those who refuse vaccines, but not NY as far as I know. temp today 98.6

Journal o the lague years, Day 685. I got my com uter ixed today. A an was making noise and had to be re laced. The an is working ok but you can see that the so twear isn't. I'm not in the mood to call tech su ort right now so this ost will be brie . As Rosanne Rosanadana used to say on SNL, "It's always something, i it's not a an, it's so tware. I it's not so tware it's an andemic. Right now I see two letters missing but I'll have to look closer and see what else is messed u . In a way it's nice. I com uter roblems were the worst thing I had to worry about, I'd be very ha y. tem today. 98.1

Journal o the lague Years, Day 686. The bad news is that my com uter is still broken. the good news is that there isn't much to re ort. The ongoing omicron variety still runs loose, but the new BA.2 varient doesn't seem much worst. I have nothing rom the grassroots to re ort, and everything either is stable or is already in the mainstream news. Is covid becoming routine? Is it going to become an endemic chronic annual surge, like the annual in luenze, or will it have variations like we have seen already? No new mutants will make covid routine, new variants can have all sorts o roblems. we'll see. tem today 97.7

Journal o the lague Years, Day 687. Yes, my little toy is still not working right. But, a tiny bit o news today. I had a routine medical visit today near enn Station on 32nd street. I walked through enn Station and counter about ten olice. All were wearing masks, most o them actually correctly. I didn't see them ticketing anyone, or doing much o anything exce t hanging around. But, there were a lot o them and a lot o masks. Maybe when they get used to wearing them on their own chins they will start en orcing the rules on others. It's not a big thing, but a tiny move in the right direction is still a tiny move in the right direction. I'll take what we can get. tem today 98.6

Journal o the lague Years, Day 691, Tuesday ebruary 22. I'm waiting or the Dell com uter eo le to come and ix my keyboard. They are waiting or an item which they need to arrive rom who knows where. Is this art o the su ly chain slowdown? I don't know, but I do know it's a ain in the ass. I have emails and articles I want to write but can't do it very easily without two letters (the one a ter "e" and the one a ter "o"). I I were really creative and had a better mastery o English maybe I could write without these letters. Maybe start a whole new genre o writing. Or maybe just have an individual quirk like bell hooks not using ca ital letters in her name. I the su ly chain allows, my com uter will be intact in the next ew days. meanwhile, tem today 98.3

Journal o the lague Year, Day 692. Another casualty o covid. NY Chemists was a small drug store on Christo her street which closed last week. I have been using them or the last ew years so I knew the owners and liked the service. I went over on Saturday to say goodbye and one o the owners ex lained. It was always hard when a small drug store tries to com ete with Rite Aide or CVS, both o which are in walking distance o NY Chemists. The drug management organizations control much o drug ricing and they requently reimbursed the store or less than their costs. All this was bad, but covid was worse. The loyal customers that allowed the store to kee in the black sto ed coming in big enough numbers to make a di erence. They held out or a while, running in the red, but eventually it became im ossible. Almost all small businesses in NYC run on small margins and covid ushed a lot over the edge, not just restaurants and bars. Some, like NY Chemists, will never come back. tem today 98.3

Journal o the lague Years, Day 693. Look at the ost by Maria Migiorini Cintron about how a customer at her restaurant hit her in the eye with a wine glass because her order wasn't out ast enough, in a very busy night at their very small restaurant. Has covid made us all crazy, or were we like this be ore and it just made it more obvious? Also, how much covid damage can occur be ore more small businesses go under? Yesterday I talked about covid hel ing to kill a small drug store. Maria and her brother are tough and one jerk customer won't get them to close their restaurant, but I wonder how many other restaurant/bars have closed because o crazy or dangerous working conditions. Some o my atients are mentally ill, but at least they're all medicated and so are little risk o ushing me into retirement too soon. tem today 97.9

Journal o the lague Years, Day 694. Yesterday in the subway I saw something or the irst time. A middle aged guy was sitting on the wooden seat with his head down looking dejected and de ressed. Two co s were about ten eet away (both wearing their masks!) and a young man and women were standing over the de ressed guy. The man had a cli board in his hand and was writing something down. The woman was talking to the guy saying something like "...we'll get you back to the residence." I went over to the women and asked her whether this was the new initiative Adams announced to get mentally ill out o the subways. She said she had been doing this or 6 years (starting way be ore covid) and worked or a non roit organization whose name I didn't catch. I've never seen these outreach workers in action in all my subway rides, but it was very good to see them now. Maybe I'll see more o them in the uture, I ho e. tem today 98.7

Journal o the lague Years, Day 697, Monday ebruary 28. With all the news rom Ukraine it might seem that there is nothing new with covid. But, there has been news. Mask mandates are being eliminated in both schools and businesses. These haven't all kicked in yet, but that being said, what is actually occurring? Walking around the West Village today I noticed some things. Workers in most stores are almost all still wearing masks, as are almost all bicycle delivery men. Many customers going into stores are wearing masks when they go in. On the street most are not wearing masks, but maybe a third are still wearing them, including me. The end o mask mandates will roll out over the next ew weeks, although there is some resistance, es ecially with kids. I'll try and be as observant as I can and let you all know. We'll see. tem today 98.3

Journal o the lague Years, Day 698. I try not to ost about something rom another medium but I saw something in a medical journal worth mentioning. A study o about 150,000 US Veterans who had covid were ollowed or a year and their history o cardiac disease was looked at. All cardiovascular diseases they looked at (heart attacks, stroke, heart ailure, etc,) had increased rates or eole who reviously had covid. No matter what the level o covid was, there were increases. So, even with mild covid there can be long term consequences. And this is just one organ system. What about the brain, kidneys, liver and, o course, the joints that are hit with arthritis when in lammation occurs. Long covid might be worse than we thought, and the need to revent covid, even the mildest cases, is still needed. Every single case. tem today 98.3

Journal o the lague Years, Day 698. About ten days ago a new initiative was started to get homeless or mentally ill individuals out o the subways. Two weeks is a short time to judge, but here are some initial observations. Last week I saw our subway riders lying down on the seats, three at 9 AM, one at 5 M. I assume they were homeless or ill, although only one o them was surrounded by a cart and bundles. There were co s scattered around at the stations. This week I saw nobody, no homeless, no co s. Did the new initiative actually work or is it too early to tell? On day 694 I described some outreach workers talking to a de ressed looking individual and trying to aid him. The unanswered question then and now is where do these individuals go when they are chased out o the subway? We'll see i Adams can increase the homes and services these eole need. That will be the real test o whether this initiative is working. tem today 98.5

Journal o the lague Years, Day 699. Yesterday I wondered where the homeless went when kicked out o the subways. Today I was walking through enn station to get Amtrek tickets. My walk through reminded me that there have been homeless in enn station or a long time. I've read that they are even more obvious and numerous late night. As I walked around the station I noticed lots o homeless scattered around the station, so the u grade rom the underground enn station to the new Moynihan has not eliminated homeless olks there. This is because we haven't solved this crises o homelessness around the city. I don't know i any o this is related to covid, which is the main theme o these osts. More detailed studies are needed to see i covid made homelessness worse or better or what. They either have been done and I missed them in the mainstream media or medical journals, or they haven't been done. I anyone has seen studies that I missed, lease ost them. When we see the size o the crises maybe that will hel us deal with it better, or maybe we'll just ignore it like be ore. tem today 98.0

Journal o the lague Years, Day 700. Almost two years with these messages, you can see my com uter is breaking down with missing with my keyboard missing letters. Be ore I break down, maybe two years is enough. On March 31 I will have done this two years exactly. Have things quieted down? I've been able to work throughout this whole andemic, have stayed healthy and use ul. The numbers o new cases in NYC is less than 2% although there are a hand ull o other states that insist on kee ing the andemic going by not getting vaccines. My own good luck, and it is luck somewhat, is holding. That's the best news I can think o at the end o the week. Three more weeks and we'll see i this should kee going or i it needs to kee going. Let's ho e there isn't another mutant coming. An endemic virus is bad news, but it's a lot better than an active andemic. I ho e. tem today 98.9

Journal o the lague Years, Day 703, Monday ebruary 7. Coming home a ter dinner last night I asked the taxi driver my usual question, "How's business?" In the ast drivers would usually say something equivocal like "good and bad" or "maybe a little better" or something like that. Last night the driver was immediate and unequivocal "O ening u " (that letter is still not working on my keyboard, sorry). Maybe he was just a very o timistic guy, or maybe just a good night, but it struck me how clear he was while all the others were unsure and tentative. Today, the mandatory checking vaccine cards ends, so maybe this is a turning oint. And maybe the good news about restaurants and bars will eventually included other jobs, schools, etc. and the hos itals (and morgues) will inally take a rest. tem today 97.8

Journal o the lague Years, Day 704. Tomorrow I leave NYC to go to a live medical convention in Baltimore. The last live convention was in November 2019 in Austin Texas. I haven't been to Baltimore is about 30 years so this will be interesting. Seeing colleagues live instead o by Zoom will also be great. I had to make sure I had the right vaccine ID or Amtrak and also the Hilton Hotel and the Convention center. I think I have everything and I ho e I don't get stranded down there with inadequate ID. I won't be osting when I'm down there but I will be back on Monday 3/14. The convention is

AMDA, the American Medical Directors Association and I will be meeting with medical directors rom nursing homes and other assisted living acilities. Also,, Dell is going to make another try to re air my com uter so maybe next week these messages will have all the letters without ga s. tem today 98.1

Journal o the lague Years, Day 710, Monday March 14. Last night I got back to NYC a ter going to a medical convention in Baltimore. It was really good to meet colleagues in erson, and not over Zoom. When sessions were done we could go to the s eakers and get or give more in ormation. I made lots o contacts I would not have made i we were over Zoom where the end o the session is really the end o the sessions. And, the 3 rece tions in the evenings were a chance to talk to others in even more detail. In general it was really enjoyable and roductive. I didn't get to see much o Baltimore other than a local ale house, but you can't have everything. I have another one in Orlando in May and Indiana olis, Indiana in November. Everyone wore masks to the sessions, everyone was vaccinated, so I ho e this meeting with 750 attendees doesn't bite us in the ass with new covid cases. I let you know in a week or so whether I caught a bug down there. One more return to normal, I think. tem today 97.9

Journal o the lague Years, Day 711. The convention I went to, besides being a good learning event, also gave a little clue as to what might be coming with other meetings. Everyone had to show vaccine cards to get in. The meeting schedule o sessions was not in a rinted book, as usual, but entirely in a hone a . It took time or me to learn it but the sta at the convention walked me through it and it eventually became easy (and easier than carrying a thick rogram.) In the sessions, everyone wore masks at virtually all times. In the rece tions, almost nobody wore masks while eating, drinking, talking, and dancing. I have two more conventions this year, and i they both work the same way it will be ok. My last live convention was 2.5 years ago, so some change was inevitable, and or the better. tem today 97.6

Journal o the lague Year, Day 712. Over the next day or two I will try and get the most ositive news rom where I work. But, meanwhile, a warning. I try not to quote the Times but they had an article today about how some good covid news had turned very bad in the Netherlands and Hong Kong. No matter how good things look, it doesn't take much to turn bad. Well, at least no new deadly variants, yet. But, things are getting better and stabilizing, at least at the level I can see at work and at the national level. Not much more to say right now, but not much more to say is actually a good thing. More good things over the next several days. tem today 97.6

Journal o the lague Years, Day 713. Although new variants are threatening in Holland and Hong Kong, things here have gotten back to normal. Almost. My assisted living acility still has some reminders. They take the tem erature o everyone entering the building. There are grou activities again in the lobby, activity room, library and dining room. But the seats are several eet away rom each other. Not 6', but still not side by side. We still wear masks when seeing residents, usually. Hurricane Ida looded our basement and it's still not re aired. These measures to limit all airway diseases might be good next year during the winter, so we've learned a little through all this. And there isn't the daily air o dread around everyone all the time. That's the best we can do right now, but that's still very good. tem today 97.8

Journal o the lague Years, Day 714. A while back I wrote about covid destroying a lot o businesses including the shoe shine store in enn Station. I went there and one guy and one women were there working a totally em ty store. Today, I went back or a shine. There were 3 or 4 women shining shoes, a guy behind the counter and another guy in the back room doing shoe re air work. My boot black (is that the right word?) had her 3 year old daughter near by laying but where she could see her at all times. The lace was busy and didn't look em ty at all. They looked like they are thriving. Many laces have survived by the skin o their teeth and are now growing and making u or lost time. Very encouraging! tem today 98.1

Journal of the Plague Years, Day 719, Wednesday March 23. (I'm writing this from work, my home computer died and is being fixed. I missed a few days posts.) Over the weekend I had brunch with 8 friends at the Ukrainian East Village Restaurant. It was for solidarity with them, but also to get together without Zoom. The covid tie-in? Virtually all the customers were maskless, even when not eating but just talking, and all of the servers were masked. So, one foot was in the return to normalcy and the other foot was still being careful. Overall numbers look good, at least in the USA. This month is two years since this started here, two really miserable years. We might be coming close to the end and I might be coming close to the end of these posts. I'll let you know in a week. no temp today, I don't have my thermometer handy. I'll try and plan better tomorrow.

Journal of the Plague Years, Day 720. I've always asked taxi drivers "how's business" during covid to see if that's an accurate view of the city from the ground view. Sunday at 5 my driver said it was slow or quiet. Last night at 10 my driver said it was pretty good and picking up. So, it looks like my attempt to use taxi drivers as information sources might not be working. Either there's too much variability from night to night or neighborhood to neighborhood, or maybe drivers themselves vary from optimist to pessimist too much. Same with the subways, too much variation from day to day. Well, I'll still try and see if there are trends, but if there are they will not be crystal clear. What is clear? Tests. See you tomorrow.

Journal of the Plague Years, Day 721. Sitting here at work, reviewing some more good news. 3 days ago the staff and residents at my alf were tested for covid. Every one was negative. Great! The more routine and downright boring these tests and precautions become, the better. I'm getting close to wrapping up these posts since next Friday will be two years of doing them. Better to wrap up on a high point than wait for something bad to happen and end up repeating stuff I've been saying for the last two years. Let's see if this next week can stay quiet.

Journal of the Plague Years, Day 725, Tuesday March 29th. At the start of this epidemic there was a race between the spread of the virus and the availability of vaccines. Now the race is between a possible second booster (the fourth jab) and the BA.2 variant, or whatever variant will come next. The epidemic is becoming more routine, like the annual flu, except more deadly. As people get used to this routing, will the fight over who is vaxxed vs un-vaxxed continue every year also? As this acute epidemic evolves into a chronic (annual?) epidemic how will be handle it? If the annual flue vaccinations are any indication, we will get used to it and simply put up with the tens or hundreds of thousands of dead every year. At least, that's the way it will be until the scientists working on a universal anti-covid vaccine are successful.

Journal of the Plague Years, Day 726. The next few days posts will be about getting back to normal. Today, I tried to get back to Burning Man which I've gone to 5 times. I was on the website, waiting for sales to open at 3 PM EST but when they did open I couldn't even get into the waiting line. I tried many times until the final announcement that "the main sale is over". This is getting back to normal in a sad way. I'd like to get back out there at least once before the big sleep but I'm slow with tech stuff and have failed at buying tickets the last few attempts. Back to normal, in a bad way. Maybe next year I'll get out there. I have to ask around to see if there's some way a boomer can expedite this.

Journal of the Plague Years, Day 728 (it should be day 730 but I miscounted somewhere). When this started two years ago, all we heard about was people fleeing the city, But, like during the fiscal crises of the 70s, the crime waves of the 80s and 90s, 9/11, Hurricane Sandy and all the other events that predicted the end of NYC people are now moving back in droves. I was listening to the Stoller report, a talk show among real estate people that's on the CUNY station 75 on Spectrum, and things have changed. The red hot market in the Hamptons of two years ago has now declined to a trickle according to them. The NYC housing market is now hot and getting hotter. NYC residents are moving back as many people, my self included, fully expected them to do. As the people move back, the city revives. Maybe not the exact same way, but one way or another it will bloom again. I've tried to use Friday for good news posts, and this is the best one I can think of.

I also think it's time to wrap up this little journal. With two years of constant posts, I've tried to present a ground level view of what's happening here that you might not always get from the mainstream media. So, for now, I'll say goodbye. The pandemic isn't completely over, so I may have to add an addendum here or there in the future. But, I'll try to limit myself with two new rules. First, I'll post about things that are new and significant and not just small permutations of existing events. Second, I'll post if I have something unique to say and not just a comment on mainstream stories. Let's hope no new posts are needed, we've all have enough.